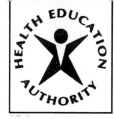
HEALTH EDUCATION AUTHORITY

Childhood immunisation: a review

Volume 1

on or before

Helen Bedford
Research Fellow
Department of Epidemiology and Public Health
Institute of Child Health
London

David Elliman
Consultant in Community Child Health
St George's Healthcare NHS Trust
London

ACKNOWLEDGEMENTS

This immunisation review owes much to the many people whose hard work and help have made it possible. We are very grateful to Dr David Salisbury and Nick Adkin at the Department of Health for their advice, guidance and input; to Plain English Campaign for their contribution; to the reviewers; and to the Health Education Authority's Immunisation Team who have all given their full support.

Health Education Authority
Trevelyan House
30 Great Peter Street
London
SW1P 2HW

Printed in England

ISBN 0 7521 0645 7

Contents

Foreword

Ten years ago, immunisation coverage in this country was amongst the lowest third of European countries. Measles epidemics were common with as many as 100,000 reported cases and up to 20 deaths in any one year. Now, coverage is amongst the highest in Europe. New vaccines have been introduced, for example Hib vaccine, with the virtual disappearance of the invasive infections caused by that organism. Epidemics are anticipated and prevented. As we go into the twenty-first century, we can look forward to the global eradication of poliomyelitis, the successful achievement of which will mean that we no longer need to immunise our children against that disease. Measles eradication might follow and with the rapid advances in molecular biology, we can expect new and improved vaccines against infectious and non-infectious diseases.

Whilst there have been considerable operational and technical improvements in immunisation over the last decade, we depend on committed and informed health professionals providing an outstanding service to parents and children. For that service to be most effective, health professionals need to be able to counsel parents in a way that is informative without being patronising, clear and concise, yet taking account of the complex issues that are involved. They must be eloquent in conveying the outstanding personal benefit that children gain through being immunised and the infinitesimally small risks that are attached. In order to undertake this task, health professionals need to understand the tensions that parents face in coming to their decisions. These three volumes provide a detailed account that helps in understanding the factors that contribute to that decision-making process, ranging from the sources of information that are available, to a full enquiry into the circumstances that have contributed to the decisions of a small, but vocal, part of the community to decline immunisation for their children. Within these volumes, the reader will achieve further insight into the interplay between health professional and parent. There will be many important messages.

Those health professionals working in immunisation have much for which they can be rightly proud. With their contribution, we have one of the leading immunisation programmes in the world. Nonetheless, we cannot afford to be complacent and must continually question if the service that we provide is the best possible. The material in these volumes will assist in that task.

DR D M SALISBURY MB BS FRCPCH MFPHM
Head, Immunisation and Infectious Diseases Group
Department of Health, London

1. Introduction: the immunisation decision

For many parents, deciding whether or not to have their child immunised can be difficult. In order to make an informed choice, you need to have accurate, balanced information about the benefits and the risks of immunisation. At the moment there is a great deal of conflicting and confusing information. This is partly because the field of immunisation is developing rapidly. New vaccines and an increasing amount of research have led to changes in knowledge about immunisation and advice about contraindications (that is, medical reasons why a vaccine should not be given) over a relatively short time. There has also been an increase in the number of non-medical people offering advice on the subject (through groups such as JABS; and publications like *The informed parent*; *What doctors don't tell you*).

In Britain, more people than ever before are having their children immunised. The benefit of immunisation is clear – fewer people develop the diseases and so fewer people suffer from serious illness or die as a result of it. Diseases such as diphtheria and polio are now extremely rare, and measles is much less common than it was only five years ago. Ironically, it is this widespread reduction in the diseases that may have led to a situation where people question the need to immunise their children. When there is less personal experience of the harmful effects of a disease and the threat of contracting the disease seems to be low, the benefits of immunising a child may not always be obvious. The possible risks of immunisation then gain more attention than the effect of the disease it protects against.

When considering certain aspects of immunisation we will look at the main issues that concern parents. This report is intended for health professionals and for parents who want more information than is provided in the *Guide to childhood immunisations*.[1] Detailed information about the signs and symptoms of diseases and reasons for and against particular vaccines are not included in this report as that information is provided in *Immunisation against infectious disease* (the 'Green book').[2]

Over the past few years a number of publications,[3-7] articles in the press[8-10] and material produced by non-medical organisations (The Informed Parent; JABS) have concentrated mainly on the possible harmful effects of immunisation. In this review, we will consider some of the issues that these publications have raised in the light of the scientific knowledge we have available. We do not claim to have all the answers, but it is important that some of the concerns raised in other publications are put into context and clarified. The scientific papers we refer to in this review have all been reviewed by other scientists and health professionals and are all available to the public.

2. Immunity

THE IMMUNE SYSTEM

In this section, we briefly describe some aspects of the immune system that are particularly relevant to immunisation. Although we know a great deal about the workings of this complex system, there is still much that is not understood.

The immune system is a complex network of cells and organs that work together to defend the body against attacks by 'foreign invaders'. These invaders are mainly organisms (that is, living structures), such as bacteria, viruses, parasites and fungi, that cause infection. The immune system can tell the difference between our own cells and those of foreign invaders. When our bodies detect something foreign, they trigger an immune response. Anything that triggers this immune response is called an **antigen**.

In rare situations, the immune system loses its ability to tell the difference between our own and foreign cells. This results in **auto immune** disease. Some forms of arthritis and diabetes are examples of this. The immune system may also react inappropriately to a foreign substance (antigen) that is usually harmless, such as dust mites or pollen. The result is an allergy and the antigens that cause the reaction are then called **allergens**.

The immune system includes a variety of cells with different functions (for example **lymphocytes**, one of the main types of immune cells; and **phagocytes** which take foreign cells into the body and destroy them). The main types of lymphocyte are B cells and T cells. B cells work mainly by releasing **antibodies**. (Antibodies are proteins which the blood produces when antigens are present.) The antibodies combine with the antigens and make them harmless. The first time B cells meet an antigen it takes some time for them to produce antibodies. But the next time they meet the same antigen, their response is much quicker because the immune system has 'remembered' the antigen.

T cells activate cell responses that are specific to a certain antigen. The first time they meet an antigen, they produce phagocytes that are not specific to the particular antigen. However, they remember the particular antigen and when the T cells meet that antigen again the cells produce lymphocytes that are specific to that antigen.

Antibodies belong to a group of proteins known as **immunoglobulins**. There are five different types of immunoglobulins, each with a different function. The five types are IgA, IgD, IgE, IgG and IgM.

As well as the responses of the B and T cells, there is also a **mucosal immune system** in the mucous membranes which line the lungs, gut and so on. This needs to be triggered separately.

IMMUNITY FROM THE MOTHER

In the last three months of pregnancy, some antibodies are passed from the mother to the unborn baby. This gives the baby a supply of antibodies from the mother's blood. The types and amounts of these antibodies vary depending on the antibodies in the mother's blood. If the mother is immune to a disease, the antibodies she has are transferred to the baby. Antibodies to whooping cough transfer to the baby but appear to offer the baby little or no protection.[1,2] Antibodies to measles usually protect a baby for about 6 to 12 months. As antibodies are transferred in the last few months of pregnancy, premature babies have less protection than those that are born after the full term.

There is a great deal of evidence to show that breastfed babies receive protection which reduces the frequency and severity of gastro-intestinal infections, respiratory infections[3] and ear infections.[4,5] The extent to which breast milk protects against other infections is unclear, although some studies have shown increased protection against *Haemophilus influenzae* type b (Hib) infection[6] (see page 42).

The protective effect may be a result of the child being exposed to fewer foreign cells as well as to the properties of the milk. There are several protective factors in breast milk, including the five types of antibody previously mentioned. In particular, IgA antibodies have an important function in limiting the way foreign cells bind to the intestinal tissue and they may also reduce the cells' ability to multiply in the gut. Other components in the milk also activate the immune system and provide protection in a number of ways.[7-9]

Interference with antibodies transferred from the mother

Antibodies which a mother passes to her baby may interfere with how the child produces antibodies after certain immunisations. So vaccines affected in this way, such as the measles, mumps and rubella vaccine (MMR), are not given until the child is 1 year old, when the antibodies from the mother have disappeared.[10]

HEALTH, IMMUNITY AND INFECTIOUS DISEASE

With a few exceptions, for example tuberculosis (TB), the health of a person exposed to a disease usually has little to do with whether or not they get the disease.[11] Malnutrition and other infections being present can make someone more likely to suffer the complications of a disease, but not change their risk of getting the disease.

For most of the common infectious diseases, the most important factor in determining whether a person will become infected is whether that person is immune. Before immunisation was introduced, nearly all children had measles and whooping cough. However, with widespread immunisation the situation is different. High rates of measles attacks happen when measles enters unvaccinated groups which may previously have been protected by the high immunisation rates in the general population (this is known as **herd immunity**). This was demonstrated in the USA when an outbreak of measles occurred among the mainly unvaccinated and susceptible Amish community. The Amish are one of the groups in the USA which refuse immunisation for religious or philosophical reasons. It could be argued that, although the Amish lifestyle is simple, it is not disadvantaged and their nutrition is good.[12] Similarly, there have been outbreaks of polio among unvaccinated religious communities in the USA and the Netherlands. A virtually identical strain of the wild polio virus that caused the outbreak in the Netherlands was also isolated from members of a community in Canada that has direct contact with the affected community.[13] Good nutrition and lifestyle alone will not prevent vulnerable people from contracting diseases like measles, and cannot completely guarantee that severe disease will not occur. In industrialised countries such as the UK, where most people have enough food, it is not clear what is the best diet for avoiding the complications of disease and whether this may differ from one person to another. Deaths and complications from disease occur even in the richer countries. Between 1970 and 1983 over half the deaths associated with measles in England and Wales occurred in previously healthy children.[14]

In malnourished populations, serious illness and death associated with infectious diseases appear to be due to low immunity caused by malnutrition. However, malnutrition tends to go hand in hand with overcrowding, poverty, poor education and poor housing; so it is difficult to isolate its effect from these other risk factors.[15] The situation is further complicated as there is no agreed definition of malnutrition.

McTaggart (1996) suggested that parents might be better off giving their children carrot juice (which is a good source of vitamin A) rather than giving them some immunisations.[16] This suggestion was based on studies in non-industrialised countries where severe vitamin A deficiency among children is a major public health problem. Vitamin A levels in the blood are further reduced during an attack of measles. This is associated with increased sickness and death rates. Trials have been carried out in countries where children with measles were given vitamin A supplements. The trials showed a clear reduction in the severity of the disease and the number of deaths.[17] However, this finding is not very relevant to children in the UK. It is well recognised that vitamin A plays an important role in the immune system, but severe vitamin A deficiency is not generally a problem in the UK. Also, there is no evidence to show that giving vitamin A supplements to children who do not have a lack of it improves the outcome of having measles. Too much vitamin A can cause damage to the liver and other organs.

It has been suggested that measles is important in the development of children and that the disease helps the immune system develop.[18,19] It has also been suggested that, after an illness, children improve physically and mentally (*personal communication* – Salli Rose, homeopath). Many practitioners of alternative medicine believe that measles helps to clear a child's system of 'toxins that built up before they were born'.[20]

There is no evidence that this is the case. Nor is there any evidence that children develop more quickly or are healthier after having measles. Once a child has recovered from a serious infection like measles, they may appear to be more energetic compared with the way he or she was before and during the illness. It is in fact well recognised that, after a bout of measles, there is a period where the child has reduced immunity. This period can last from several weeks to several years. During this time a child is at risk from other infections.[21] This is particularly evident in non-industrialised countries where children have a higher risk of dying after a bout of measles compared with children who have been immunised against measles. A study in West Africa showed that after three years, children who had suffered measles infection had lower general immunity than vaccinated children who had not had measles.[22]

IMMUNISATION – PASSIVE AND ACTIVE

Immunity may follow a natural infection (either with symptoms or without symptoms) or after immunisation. Immunisation is the process by which a person artificially gets protection against a disease or its complications without being exposed to the natural infection. You can get immunity by active or passive immunisation.

Passive immunisation

Antibodies are injected into the body. The immune system is not stimulated to produce its own antibodies, so passive immunisation provides immediate protection but only for a few weeks or months.

Active immunisation

A vaccine is introduced into the body either by mouth or by injection. Vaccines contain organisms which may be either live but weakened, so they are not able to cause the full-blown illness, or killed. Many viral vaccines, such as those for measles, mumps and rubella, contain live (but weakened) viruses. The standard whooping cough vaccine contains the killed (inactivated) organism. More recently, some vaccines (such as that for hepatitis B) have been produced using genetic engineering.

The antigens contained in vaccines stimulate the immune system to produce specific antibodies as though it had been exposed to a natural infection. This presents little or no risk to the person receiving the vaccine. Immunity develops as a result of the immune system's memory. If the same antigen then enters the body through natural infection, the immune system is already primed to fight the disease by immediately producing specific antibodies. A certain level of immunity is necessary to make sure the vaccinated person remains protected against disease. On the whole, vaccines containing live organisms give longer-lasting immunity. Some vaccines provide long- lasting protection, while others must be repeated at intervals.

Vaccine effectiveness

The effectiveness of a vaccine is judged by evidence that it protects against the natural disease. Although the production of antibodies is often only an indirect measure of protection, it is frequently a good guide. In some cases, for example in whooping cough, the immune response that provides protection is not clearly understood and high concentrations of antibodies do not always mean good protection.

Sometimes, a particular person does not become immune after receiving a vaccine. This is known as **primary vaccine failure** and there may be many reasons for it. The vaccine may have been stored at the incorrect temperature and may therefore have become ineffective. In the case of MMR, the vaccine may have been given while the child was too young, so its effect was cancelled by the antibodies the child got from his or her mother. Or it may simply not 'take' for no apparent reason.

Secondary vaccine failure occurs when a vaccine provides immunity at first, but then that immunity disappears.

Herd immunity

Immunisation protects not only the individual but also the community. When enough people are immunised, the disease is less likely to be transferred from one person to another and so there is less disease in the community as a whole. With infectious diseases such as measles, diphtheria, whooping cough and polio, the unimmunised are protected by the immunity of the majority. This is referred to as herd immunity. The percentage of individuals in a population who need to be immunised in order to create herd immunity varies with the effectiveness of the vaccine and the characteristics of the disease.

No vaccine is 100% effective, which means that a small number of people who receive a vaccine will not be fully protected. There is also variation in the effectiveness of different vaccines. For example, measles vaccine is 90–95% effective. So if 100 children are given the vaccine, between 5 and 10 of them will not be protected against the disease. Measles has been described as the most infectious organism known to man. In order to create a herd immunity to measles infection, at least 95% of the population need to receive the vaccine.[23]

This does not mean that vaccines do not work but that, in some cases they do not provide complete protection. When someone in this situation gets an infection the disease is often less severe. In a survey of 8000 cases of whooping cough, Miller and Fletcher (1976) found that a few fully-vaccinated children got the disease.[24] However, when the severity of disease (in terms of the number of complications) was compared between the vaccinated and unvaccinated groups, it was found that vaccination reduced the severity of the disease. No fully-immunised child has died from whooping cough in the UK.

The most effective way of protecting people who do not respond to the vaccine and those who cannot be given them for medical reasons (such as children with impaired immunity) is by herd immunity. This is achieved by making sure most of the population receives the vaccine.

CONTENTS OF VACCINES

Vaccines may contain the following substances.

Active immunising antigens

Active immunising antigens include killed, intact bacterium (eg whole-cell whooping cough vaccine); live (but weakened) viruses (eg oral polio, measles, mumps, rubella vaccine); inactivated bacterial toxins (eg diphtheria and tetanus toxoids); and purified bacterial sugars (polysaccharides) (eg Hib vaccine).

In the case of live vaccines, the organism may be grown in different ways. Rubella vaccines are grown in a cell culture called MRC5. This cell culture was developed in the 1960s from a small number of cells taken from a single fetus (where the fetus had been aborted on medical grounds). The rigorous purification process during manufacturing removes all traces of the cells the vaccine is grown in, so that there is no fetal tissue or fetal cells in the vaccine. The measles and mumps components of MMR are grown in cell cultures from chicken eggs, and individuals who have a history of extreme reaction to eggs should be given MMR vaccine only under closeobservation.[25,26]

Suspending fluid

Some vaccines are suspended in a fluid. This may be sterile water or salt water, or it may be a complex tissue-culture fluid containing protein or other constituents from the medium in which the vaccine is produced.

Preservatives, stabilisers and antibiotics

Extremely small amounts of chemicals and certain antibiotics are often necessary to prevent bacteria growing or to stabilise the antigen. Many vaccines contain thiomersal, a compound which contains mercury and prevents contamination. Although rare allergic reactions have occurred, there have never been any other toxic reactions relating to it.

Adjuvants (substances which increase the body's immune response to an antigen)

An aluminium compound is often used to improve the body's response to the vaccine.

Although accumulations of aluminium have been found in the brains of patients with Alzheimer's Disease, there is no evidence that aluminium causes the disease.[27] Also, there is no evidence that aluminium hydroxide given as a component of a vaccine has any long-term adverse effects.[28,29] However, newer adjuvants are being investigated.

If the person receiving a vaccine is sensitive to any of these constituents, they may have an allergic reaction.

3. Information about immunisation

The purpose of this review is to examine some concerns and issues about immunisation in the light of the scientific evidence available. So it is important to consider the sources of information about the need for immunisation – its risks, benefits and effects.

Before any vaccine is introduced, the need to prevent a disease must be shown by medical information about the pattern, frequency and age group affected, together with information about associated severe illness and death, and whether the disease can be treated. Meningococcal meningitis is a disease that is relatively uncommon (compared with, for example, measles before widespread immunisation), but its associated severity and high death rate make its prevention highly desirable.

The number of cases of a disease may differ from country to country. This is partly because of different reporting systems, but real differences have been found in, for example, the incidence of Hib disease not only between countries, but also between populations within the same country.[1] Microbiological investigation is also important. Meningococcal disease may be caused by one of a number of different strains of an organism. In England and Wales the organisms from patients with meningococcal disease are examined by the Meningococcal Reference Unit (MRU) to monitor patterns of the disease. Type B is the commonest strain in this country.[2]

In this country information about deaths is collected through the Office for National Statistics. Information about the complications associated with a particular disease is not routinely collected, but reliable information is gathered from surveys.

PRE-LICENSING EVALUATION OF VACCINE EFFECTIVENESS AND SAFETY

Before any vaccine is licensed for use, its safety and effectiveness must be proved. Trials of vaccines are designed to measure antibody response, their effectiveness at protecting against disease, and the nature and frequency of vaccine reactions. Trials of a new vaccine are carried out in three phases.[3]

Phase I

Vaccine is given to a small number of healthy adult volunteers to show that it does not cause any serious or unexpected side effects.

Phase II

These trials are usually done with a sample of 100 to 200 people for whom the vaccine is intended. Antibody responses to the vaccine are measured, as are the nature and frequency of more common reactions. This information is compared with a group of people who are not receiving the vaccine. A study of the safety and immunogenicity (the ability to produce an immune response) of a combined diphtheria, tetanus, whooping cough and Hib vaccine included 378 children, who were chosen at random to receive either a combined vaccine or separate vaccines. In these types of trials it is common for parents to record information about side effects.[4]

Phase III

Protection against disease is evaluated by comparing the number of vaccinated and unvaccinated people who get the disease. A vaccine is considered effective if it *significantly* reduces the disease incidence in the immunised group compared with that seen in the unvaccinated group.

ROUTINE TESTING OF VACCINES BEFORE RELEASE

Each batch of vaccine goes through extensive quality control and safety testing before it is released for general use. This is to make sure that each dose is safe, pure and potent enough to be effective. Not only are strict quality controls undertaken during the process of manufacture, but each batch of vaccine is tested by both the manufacturer and an independent assessor before it is released into general use.[5]

POST-LICENSING MONITORING OF VACCINES AND VACCINATION PROGRAMMES

Once a vaccine has been licensed and is in general use, post-licensing evaluation for safety continues. Vaccines are monitored closely in order to detect any rare or new reactions that may not have been apparent in the trial situation. The effect the vaccination programme has on the target diseases also needs monitoring. This is achieved through a combination of surveillance of infectious disease through routine reports or special surveys, as well as monitoring vaccine coverage. Changes in the effectiveness of a vaccine are also monitored. Surveys may help determine the need for a change in vaccine policy. For example, studies among school children showed that the number of children who were susceptible to measles rose between 1986 to 1987 and 1991. Mathematical modelling predicted that the level of susceptibility in 1995 would have been high enough to allow a large epidemic of measles. This pointed to the need for a second dose of vaccine for the school population in order to avoid an epidemic.[6]

THE RISKS OF IMMUNISATION VERSUS DISEASE

All vaccines can cause side effects, but these are rarely severe. When deciding whether to have your child immunised, it is important to compare the risk of immunisation with the risk of the disease. Despite concerns about vaccine safety, vaccination is safer than accepting the risks for the diseases.[7]

Studies of vaccine safety

Studying the short-term and long-term consequences of immunisation is not straightforward. In any individual, coincidences between two events, such as receiving a vaccine and getting a disease, may suggest cause and effect. This can be misleading. For example, event A can happen before event B, but be totally unrelated as there may be a third factor that causes the association. Chance alone may also result in the apparent linking of events.[8] For example, some women who take iron supplements during pregnancy have children with Down's syndrome, but it is also true that some women who do not take iron supplements also have children with Down's syndrome.

To find out whether an event such as convulsions is related to a vaccination, it is essential to look at:

- a group of children who have had the vaccine;

- a group of children who are similar except that they have not had the vaccine; and

- the frequency of convulsions in both groups.

This is known as a cohort study. Case reports of events occurring among *individual* children do not provide this information, so the true frequency of these events, and therefore the risk figures, cannot be worked out.

Cohort studies are one way of detecting the risk of adverse side effects associated with immunisation. The risk can also be detected by carrying out a case-control study. In a case-control study (which is better than a cohort study at investigating rare events), histories of vaccination are gathered from patients with a specific condition that is possibly related to vaccination. These are then compared to a group of **controls** who do not have the condition, but are of a similar age and the same sex.[3]

This approach to finding out whether adverse events are associated with immunisation is particularly important, since most vaccines are given to children in the first year of life. As this is a time when it is not uncommon for unrelated problems to be recognised, their diagnosis may coincide with immunisation.

REPORTING ADVERSE REACTIONS OF VACCINES

The pre-licensing evaluation of vaccines includes intense monitoring of vaccine reactions, although among fewer children than the millions who receive the vaccine once it is in general use. After a vaccine is introduced, adverse reactions continue to be monitored. In this country, health professionals are asked to report suspected adverse reactions to the Committee on Safety of Medicines, using the yellow card system. The present reporting system is voluntary. It is well recognised that this system is not ideal. Accurate surveillance of adverse reactions depends on early, complete and accurate reporting of reactions.[9] A voluntary reporting scheme means that adverse events are often not fully reported. It also means that standard criteria for reporting reactions are not used and there may not be follow-up to find out the outcome of reported reactions.[10] Also, voluntary reports cannot be used to suggest causes for events such as convulsions, which can occur without immunisation.

New, more reliable methods of monitoring adverse reactions are being investigated. One approach has only become possible since the widespread use of computers and involves linking hospital admission records with immunisation records. A study using this method found it to be reliable, and it is hoped that it will form the basis of a new national system for routinely monitoring vaccine safety.[11]

4. The effect immunisation programmes have on the incidence of infectious diseases

The introduction of vaccines, along with other public health improvements such as clean water supplies, has had a profound effect on world health. Worldwide, vaccination programmes have either prevented or significantly reduced the incidence of the major childhood infections – smallpox, polio, diphtheria, tetanus, whooping cough, measles, mumps and rubella.

HAVE IMMUNISATION PROGRAMMES WORKED?

It is often stated that the incidence of and deaths from infectious diseases had already dramatically reduced before any vaccine was used.[1] This is true. Improvements in living conditions and a reduction in overcrowding played a very important role in reducing infectious disease and its effects. But the introduction of immunisation has resulted in a further and more rapid decline in disease incidence and deaths than would have occurred through other public health measures alone. Immunisation plays an important role in controlling disease and makes it possible to completely wipe out some diseases. It is unlikely that smallpox would have been wiped out without vaccination. This has been the result of an effective immunisation programme combined with intense searching for cases and adequate public health control measures worldwide.[2] We can now eliminate other infectious diseases, such as polio, not only from industrialised countries but also from non-industrialised countries, where improvements in living conditions have been less dramatic.

The introduction of Hib vaccine to the UK in 1992 provides a powerful example of the effect an immunisation programme can have where there is no noticeable improvement in living conditions. Within one year of the vaccine being introduced there was an 80% decline in laboratory-confirmed Hib meningitis and septicaemia (blood poisoning) in children under one and by 1995 the decline was 95%.[3] A similar effect has been observed in all countries which have introduced the Hib vaccine (see page 43).

Widespread vaccination of children has had a dramatic effect on the incidence of measles and its associated complications. In England and Wales cases of measles began to be reported in 1940. Figure 1 shows the epidemic cycle of the disease, with an average of 250,000 cases reported and 80 deaths a year, and over 600,000 cases reported in a peak year. Following the introduction of immunisation in 1968, the size of measles epidemics was reduced, but vaccine uptake was never high enough to prevent epidemics altogether. However, since the MMR vaccine was introduced in 1988, uptake has been very high. This has

Figure 1 Measles notifications: cases and deaths, England and Wales 1940–93

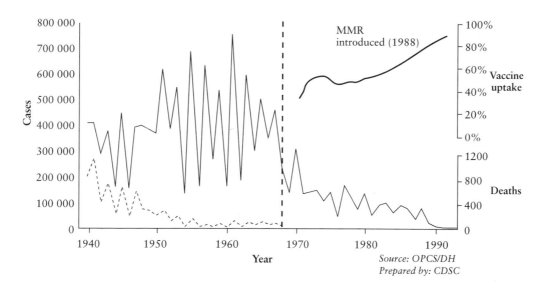

Source: OPCS/DH
Prepared by: CDSC

had a major effect on the number of cases reported, leading to several years of low measles incidence and only 11 deaths associated with the disease.[4]

Deaths from whooping cough declined in the USA, the UK and Sweden before immunisation was introduced, but there is considerable evidence to show that widespread vaccination has resulted in dramatic decreases in incidences as well as death rates. In England and Wales between 1978 and 1994, vaccine uptake increased from 31% to 93% of 2-year-olds, and the number of cases reported fell from 65,810 to 3963 between 1982 and 1994.[5] Death from whooping cough is now rare in this country. Further evidence of the value of the vaccination includes the recurrence of major outbreaks in the UK, Sweden and Japan when vaccination rates fell in the 1970s. Fears about the safety of the vaccine after reports linking it with brain damage led to whooping cough immunisation rates in England and Wales falling from 79% in 1973 to 31% in 1978 (Figure 2). In some parts of the country rates dropped to as low as 9%. This was followed by whooping cough epidemics in 1977 to 1979 and 1981 to 1983, with over 100,000 cases reported in each period and 51 deaths. The disease was commonest in areas where vaccine uptake was low.[6]

There was an epidemic of polio every year in the USA in the first half of this century. This represented a major public health problem and in the peak year of 1952 there were 21,269 cases of crippling polio. The widespread introduction of polio vaccination has led to a dramatic decline in the incidence of polio and the World Health Organization has set the goal of wiping out the disease by the year 2000. Polio has now been wiped out from the western hemisphere and other polio-free areas are also emerging.

The reduction in infectious disease since immunisation was introduced is clear evidence of the effect of immunisation programmes. However, a vaccine's effectiveness in preventing disease can only be demonstrated by comparing disease rates among immunised and unimmunised groups.

Figure 2 Pertussis: England and Wales 1940–94

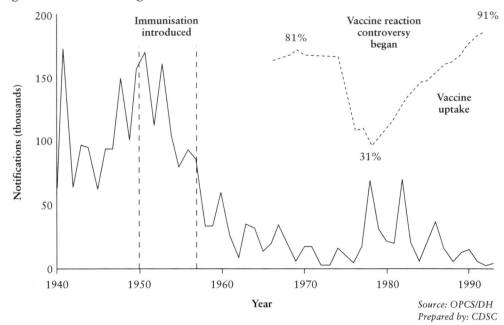

HEALTH AND FINANCIAL BENEFITS OF VACCINATION

Analyses of vaccination programmes have shown them to be valuable both in financial terms and in terms of lives saved and disability avoided. Bloch et al (1985) calculated the enormous benefits arising from the first 20 years of measles vaccination in the USA.[7] These are shown in Table 1.

Table 1 – Health and financial benefits due to vaccination against measles in the USA, 1963-1982[7]

Number of cases avoided	52 107 000
Number of lives saved	5 210
Number of cases of brain damage avoided	17 370
Number of extra years of normal and productive life resulting from preventing premature death and brain damage	1 558 000
Number of health professional visits saved	26 776 000
Number of hospital days saved	2 972 000
Savings achieved	$5 120 729 000

THE CHANGING PATTERN OF INFECTIOUS DISEASE

There has been a change in the pattern of some diseases due to the use of vaccines. When vaccine uptake is not high enough to create herd immunity, the incidence of an infection is reduced but not eliminated from the community. For vulnerable people who do not receive the vaccine, or who do not receive full protection from the vaccine, their exposure to natural infection tends to be delayed until they are older. (This is undesirable as diseases such as measles tend to be more severe in older people as well as in the very young.) This may be part of the reason for measles outbreaks among college students in the USA and was the reason for the recent MR (measles and rubella) campaign in the UK. Both these issues are discussed later in this review (see pages 31 and 37).

As well as a major decrease in the total number of cases of measles in all age groups, there has been a change in the age groups suffering from measles. The proportion of reported cases in children under one increased from 9% in 1987 to 28% in 1991.[8] This is mostly because the high uptake of MMR vaccine in the second year of life has resulted in a decrease in the number of cases of measles in older children. However, it is also known that the level of measles antibody that a woman transfers to her baby is lower and may disappear more rapidly when she has been immunised rather than having natural measles infection.[9,10] The extent to which this affects the proportion of cases in children under one is unclear. The current high levels of vaccine uptake will mean that, in the future, most mothers in the UK will have been vaccinated rather than becoming immune through natural infection. This may mean that eventually measles vaccine will be recommended for children under one.[10]

There has also been a change in the pattern of some infectious diseases for which there is currently no immunisation programme, such as chickenpox. Over the past 20 years, there has been an unexplained upward shift in the age of infection. This has important consequences. Although chickenpox is generally a mild disease in childhood, it may be life-threatening in patients with reduced immunity, normal adults, particularly pregnant women, and newborn infants when the mother had the infection close to the time of delivery.[11]

OUTBREAKS OF DISEASE AMONG OLDER AGE GROUPS AND HIGHLY-VACCINATED GROUPS

Outbreaks of disease, in particular measles, among older age groups and highly-vaccinated groups are well documented. They are sometimes used to suggest that the vaccines are ineffective.[12]

Without a vaccination programme most individuals develop immunity to measles through being exposed to the disease when they are young. When there is a high uptake of the measles vaccine, a period of low measles incidence (known as the 'honeymoon period') follows. During this time, because there is less disease in the community, natural exposure no longer occurs. Groups of vulnerable children who were not immunised in the early years of the programme or who did not respond to the vaccine can reach older ages before being exposed to measles. The number of vulnerable individuals in the community gradually grows until there are enough to cause an epidemic affecting mainly older children or young adults. Though the percentage of cases in older children increases after the introduction of vaccination, the total number of cases across all age groups falls. After high uptake of a vaccine for several years, children getting the disease are increasingly likely to be those who have not responded to the vaccine.[13]

Since no vaccine is 100% effective, when there is an outbreak of a disease there will always be some cases occurring in vaccinated individuals. In a country with no immunisation, all of the cases of whooping cough would be in children who had not been immunised. In a country where all the children are immunised, the introduction of whooping cough would result in a few cases, all of them in immunised children. If whooping cough were introduced into a school with 100 children, 90 of whom were fully immunised, 7 of the 10 unprotected children would be expected to catch whooping cough, but 1 in 10 of the immunised children (that is, 9 of the 90 immunised children) would also be expected to catch the disease. So of the total of 16 cases in the school, 9 (i.e. over half) would be children who had been immunised. It could easily be assumed that the vaccine was ineffective, but proper examination of the figures shows the vaccine to have been about 85% effective. If there had been no vaccination at the school, about 70 of the 100 children would have contracted the disease.

5. General issues

SYSTEM OF PAYING GENERAL PRACTITIONERS FOR IMMUNISATION

In 1990 a new system of paying for immunisation was introduced. Under that system general practitioners (GPs) are paid at differing levels according to the percentage of children on their practice list who are fully immunised. For example, they receive a lower payment if 70% of eligible children are immunised, and a higher payment if 90% are immunised. GPs have always been paid for immunisation although, before 1990, payment was made for each child immunised rather than the percentage immunised. This has led to the argument that health professionals are more interested in immunising as many children as possible than in parents' concerns about the benefits and risks of immunisation. There have been claims that some parents have been put under pressure to have their children immunised,[1] and findings from qualitative research support these claims.[2-4] This is a cause for concern and needs to be investigated further.

INTERESTS OF PHARMACEUTICAL COMPANIES

It has been claimed that: 'Government statistics have consistently been manipulated to "prove" the effectiveness of Government-funded inoculation procedures. Research to "prove" the effectiveness of individual inoculations has been funded by pharmaceutical companies who have a vested interest both in their sale, and also in playing down any possible damage they cause'.[1] No evidence is provided to support this claim. Although it is true that some vaccine research is funded by vaccine manufacturers, there is also a wealth of independent research. Since vaccines are given to healthy individuals, the research to investigate their effectiveness and safety is extremely rigorous. It is not in the interests of the Government or the vaccine manufacturers to falsify the effectiveness of poor vaccines, since their lack of effectiveness would soon become apparent once they were introduced into general use. Safety is always paramount. It was a Department of Health initiative to establish a monitoring system for adverse events following excess reports of aseptic meningitis associated with MMR vaccine in 1990–91.[5]

CHANGES IN IMMUNISATION SCHEDULES

In 1990 the schedule for routine immunisation in this country changed. The primary course of immunisations (diphtheria, tetanus, whooping cough and polio) previously started at 3 months of age and was completed at 10–11 months of age. The primary course now starts at 2 months and is completed at 4 months. This change was made to make sure the youngest children, who are most at risk from the severe complications of whooping cough, are protected. Also to increase coverage throughout the country by having a uniform schedule.

Studies have shown that:

- children immunised at this lower age are less likely to have reactions to the vaccines;[6,7]

- the immunisation schedule provides an adequate and immediate immune response;[8]

- the protection provided is probably enough to last until the pre-school booster;[9] and

- higher coverage is achieved earlier so more children are being protected.

CHANGES IN RECOMMENDATIONS FOR IMMUNISATION

Changes in the official guidance on immunisation, such as altering the schedule for immunisation, may lead some parents to feel that they are receiving conflicting advice – the advice they received for an older child may differ from that which they would now receive for a new baby. For example, it is now recommended that children with stable neurological conditions or well-controlled epilepsy can be immunised against whooping cough. Science develops greater certainty with time and as greater and more detailed knowledge and experience is gathered. The overall move on immunisation has been from a wisely cautious approach to a more justifiable one, as the safety and benefits of immunisation have become more and more evident.

IMMUNISATION OF PREMATURE BABIES

Premature babies are particularly vulnerable to infection and are particularly at risk from the effects of whooping cough. Studies have shown that immunisation is effective and safe in premature babies.[10-15] The date of immunisation should be calculated from the child's actual date of birth, not from expected date of delivery. This may mean that some babies are immunised while they are still in special care or neo-natal units.

6. Experiences of immunisation and infectious diseases in other countries

Immunisation practice and patterns of infectious disease in other countries can provide useful insights. However, direct comparison between countries is not always valid as few countries have such a complete system of monitoring the incidence of infectious diseases and vaccine uptake as we have in the UK. Some of the examples below have been chosen because they have been discussed in the literature produced by those who question immunisation. Most of the examples relate to whooping cough.

In both industrialised and non-industrialised countries, widespread use of vaccines has had dramatic effects. Most countries have eliminated diphtheria, polio and tetanus in the newborn. Whooping cough and measles have also shown sharp declines in incidence.[1]

SWEDEN

Dr Joanna Cleeton claimed in a newspaper that, 'Sweden doesn't have whooping cough or diphtheria jabs and their decline has been the same as in other countries'.[2] Swedish infants are given all the routine vaccines that are offered in this country, except for the whooping cough vaccine and they use an inactivated polio vaccine (that is, one containing the killed virus) instead of oral polio vaccine. A change in vaccine production methods in the early 1970s appeared to result in loss of effectiveness of the whooping cough vaccine used and so its use was discontinued in 1979. After three years with only a few cases of whooping cough, the incidence gradually increased with outbreaks in 1983 and 1985.[3] There have been some deaths associated with the complications of the disease since 1981 (*personal communication* – Dr M. Blennow). The present situation in Sweden is that prevention of the disease by general vaccination is 'urgently needed'.[3] There have been several major vaccine trials and a new whooping cough vaccine has now been introduced.

JAPAN

Experiences with whooping cough and whooping cough immunisation in Japan, Germany and Italy have been described by writers as showing that immunisation is not effective in preventing whooping cough.[4] In 1975 whooping cough immunisation was suspended for two months following the deaths of two children. They died 24 hours after receiving the whooping cough vaccine, although it was later found that their deaths were not caused by the vaccination.[5] When whooping cough vaccine was used again, it was recommended that the age for vaccination should be raised to 2 years.[6] Because 2-year-old children had already received the vaccine in their first year, acceptance rates suddenly dropped and doctors did not actively encourage vaccination. The number of whooping cough cases increased rapidly, approximately 20-fold in five years,[7] and it was found that almost all of the affected children had not been immunised or had not completed a course. This 'made it clear that whooping cough vaccine had been effective'.[6]

The Japanese then started to develop a new whooping cough vaccine and, in 1981, an acellular whooping cough vaccine was introduced. This was done without having any real information about the vaccine's effectiveness. Although there is no complete national system for reporting cases of infectious disease in Japan, information is collected through reports to the Ministry of Health and Welfare and a surveillance system of 2000 physicians and paediatricians who report the weekly number of patients with infectious diseases. After the introduction of the acellular vaccine in 1981, the uptake rate gradually increased to 85% by 1986 and reported cases of the disease and deaths from whooping cough declined. Although the vaccine was given to children over the age of 2, the incidence of whooping cough also declined in children under 2 years (although most cases were in this age group). In 1988 the Ministry of Health and Welfare announced that whooping cough immunisation could be given to infants over the age of 3 months.[8]

MMR vaccine was introduced into Japan in 1989. Some of the vaccines used contained the Urabe or similar strains of the mumps virus. Cases of post-vaccination aseptic meningitis were reported and linked to that particular vaccine virus.[9] Because the Japanese had no alternative vaccine licensed for use, MMR vaccine was withdrawn and, because they do not have a combined measles, rubella vaccine, these vaccines have continued to be given separately. In the meantime, work is going on to develop an alternative combined MMR vaccine for use in Japan.

ITALY

By law, all children in Italy must be immunised against diphtheria, tetanus, polio and hepatitis B. Children must have proof of immunisation before they can go to school. However, whooping cough, measles, mumps and rubella vaccines are only recommended, although laws are currently being considered which would make them compulsory. Uptake of the whooping cough vaccine is low at present, with only an estimated 38% of Italian children under 5 being vaccinated.[10]

Italy is one of the ten wealthiest nations in the world and the pattern of a disease such as whooping cough gives insight into its severity among a largely non-immunised population in a developed country. Epidemics continue to occur every three to five years, and approximately 25% of Italian children have had whooping cough by their fifth birthday. Whooping cough is most severe in children under one and in this group about 1 in 14 children needs to go to hospital and 1 in 850 dies. Between 1980 and 1987 there were 51 deaths from whooping cough with more than 80% of these in children under one.[10]

GERMANY

In Germany there are no national statistics on whooping cough incidence or on vaccine uptake. National immunisation policy is interpreted at a local level. Local studies have shown that whooping cough is common, with vaccine uptake as low as 7% in some areas. The general picture of whooping cough in Germany resembles the situation in the UK after the decline in vaccine uptake in the mid to late 1970s.[11]

UNITED STATES OF AMERICA

McTaggart claims that 'no form of the measles portion of the vaccine (MMR) appears to be working', and proposes that the outbreaks of measles in the USA among groups that include vaccinated individuals are evidence for this.[12] In all states in the USA, children must have proof of immunisation against infectious disease, including whooping cough, before they start school. However, parents can opt out of immunisation on ideological or religious grounds. Although no national information is collected on vaccine uptake, surveys show that the uptake rate for 5-year-olds is very high (97–98%). However, in some inner city populations, the uptake rate of measles vaccine among 2-year-olds is as low as 50%.

Although measles incidence rates were very low in the USA in the 1980s and the country was held up as a model of measles control, there was a resurgence of measles in 1989-91, with 55,622 reported cases and 166 deaths.[13] Outbreaks occurred in two main groups – vaccinated children aged 5 to 19 and, most significantly, unvaccinated pre-school children. In the second group, those living in deprived inner city areas where preventive child health services are poor were particularly affected.[14]

Studies of outbreaks among school children in the USA have found attack rates in vaccinated populations to be consistent with the expected primary vaccine failure rate (about 5%). Secondary vaccine failure has occurred, but rates appear to be low (under 0.2%).[15]

In 1989 the USA introduced a two-dose measles vaccination. Vaccine is now given at 12 to 15 months and then either at 4 to 5 years or 11 to 12 years of age. There has been a marked decline in measles incidence in the USA since 1991. In 1995 a total of 301 cases were reported, the lowest number of cases ever reported in one year since measles outbreaks were first reported in 1912.[16] Measles infections can, of course, be brought into the country from abroad.[17] As this possibility has become more obvious, it has emphasised the need for continued vaccine uptake even when there is low disease incidence.

FINLAND

The USA experience with measles shows how difficult it is to control this disease. No country has eliminated measles with one dose of the vaccine. More than 30 European countries (including Sweden and Finland) and New Zealand have adopted a two-dose vaccine schedule. Since Finland introduced a two-dose

MMR vaccine schedule in 1982 the incidence of the three diseases has been reduced by more than 90%. Indigenous ('home grown') cases of measles, mumps and rubella have been nearly wiped out of the country. There are now fewer than 30 cases of each disease every year, and these are probably imported from other countries.[18]

7. Alternatives to immunisation

A number of alternatives to immunisation have been put forward. One suggestion is to strengthen a child's immune system through a healthy diet of natural foods with hardly any chemical additives or refined products. The child would then be less susceptible to disease and better equipped to deal with it rapidly and effectively.[1] The effect of health on infectious disease was discussed earlier in this review (page 3). However, there is no scientific evidence to support this opinion.

HOMEOPATHIC VACCINES

Homeopathic vaccines have also been suggested as an alternative to conventional immunisation. However, even some homeopathic practitioners disagree about the benefit of these vaccines. They are recommended for use when a child has contact with an infectious disease, as there is no evidence to suggest that they produce long-term immunity. 'There is no basis in homeopathic theory or principle for the routine and wholesale administration of potentised substances for long-term prevention'.[2] Homeopathic medicines are prescribed for existing symptoms and it is not known what effect they could have when there is no clear need for their use. This means that they can only be used when a child is already suffering from the effects of a disease. They are unlikely to save the life of a child with meningitis.

There is also a lack of evidence to suggest they provide protection in the short term: 'There is only anecdotal evidence that homeopathic medicines are sometimes effective used in this way'.[3] Clinical studies have been attempted, but they have 'all suffered from serious methodological shortcomings'.[4]

It has been argued that it would be extremely difficult to carry out a major trial on how effective homeopathic preparations are in preventing infectious disease as the number of cases of whooping cough for example, is now so low in the UK.[3]

A pilot study was set up to examine whether the homeopathic preparation 'Pertussin 30' was effective in preventing whooping cough. The researcher admits that the methods used in the trial were unsound and so he was unable to demonstrate the usefulness of 'Pertussin 30' in preventing the disease. However, he did conclude that there were grounds for a larger study.[5]

Homeopaths' views on conventional immunisation

Opposition to immunisation is sometimes attributed to homeopaths. In fact, even among homeopathic practitioners there are differing views about immunisation. The Faculty of Homeopathy, whose members are medically qualified, recommends: 'Where there is no medical contraindication, immunisation should be carried out in the normal way using conventional tested and approved vaccines …. We do not have the research data showing the persistence of satisfactory antibody levels after using homeopathic preparations for immunisation, and this is why the advice is to use the "conventional" vaccines if at all possible.'

The Society of Homeopaths, which tends to represent lay practitioners of homeopathy, does not have an official policy on vaccination (*personal communication* – Felicity Lee). However, it believes parents should have access to information on effectiveness and safety. In 1990 the organisation published a leaflet called *Vaccination – a difficult decision*. This leaflet has been described in the *British Homeopathic Journal* as: '… painting a highly tendentious and alarmist picture of immunisation, as well as containing some fundamental scientific errors'.[4]

It is important to note that Hahnemann, the doctor who founded homeopathy, was a strong supporter of vaccination. He considered it to be 'a clear and convincing demonstration of the Law of Similitude'.[4]

EXCLUDING CERTAIN VACCINES OR DELAYING IMMUNISATION

It has been suggested that parents could choose certain vaccines for their child and delay others (for example, tetanus) until the child is older.[1] This is based on the belief that introducing a number of vaccines all together into the system of a very young child is potentially harmful and may overload the immune system, and that children are only at risk of certain infections when older.

There is no evidence that very young children are unable to cope with a number of vaccines given together. Even premature babies have been shown to have a good response to the primary vaccines.[6-8] There is no evidence that the immune system can be overloaded – the number of antigens in the routinely administered vaccines is small in comparison with the number of antigens the body faces every day. Immunising children aged 2 to 4 months has been shown to produce fewer adverse reactions than immunising them at 3 to 11 months.[9] Children are vaccinated at a young age in order to protect them when they are at their most vulnerable. Whooping cough in particular is more likely to lead to complications and death in very young babies. Giving Hib vaccine before a child is 6 months old means that the child is protected before the peak age for Hib infection (at 6 to 12 months old).

8. Specific conditions that have been claimed to be linked to immunisation

SUDDEN INFANT DEATH SYNDROME (ALSO KNOWN AS COT DEATH)

The possibility of a link between the diphtheria, tetanus and whooping cough vaccine and Sudden Infant Death Syndrome is one of the most serious of the suggested adverse effects of the vaccine.

Scheibner (1993) was involved in work in which babies' breathing was monitored and the effects of various events, such as teething and infectious disease, noted.[1] She states that the older brother or sister of some of the babies in the study had died from cot death and that the parents reported they had most commonly died after receiving the diphtheria, tetanus and whooping cough vaccine. Scheibner considers that the vaccine is a major cause of cot death.

Cot death occurs chiefly in babies between the ages of 2 weeks and 1 year. Its incidence rate changes during the first year of life, with a peak at 3 months of age. Research into the causes of cot death has identified a number of factors which increase the risk. These include, low birthweight, premature birth, multiple birth, being male, poverty, a mother who smokes, and the baby's sleeping position.[2] Research also suggests that some cases are actually due to undiagnosed whooping cough.[3]

The timing of cot death, with a peak at about three months of age, is at a time when children are receiving vaccines. This has led to the suggestion that immunisation may be the cause of some cot deaths. Much research has concentrated on investigating the possibility of such a link.

In 1989, the Institute of Medicine in the USA set up a committee to look at the adverse consequences of whooping cough and rubella vaccines. This was as part of the National Vaccine Injury Act, which established a no-fault compensation system for individuals possibly injured by vaccines.

In their report the committee point out that reports of single, or multiple cases, of SIDS deaths within hours, days or weeks of immunisation offer limited insight into the possibility of a causal relationship between the two events. This is because SIDS occurs primarily in the first year of life when babies are being immunised and so some cases of SIDS would be expected in the period following immunisation. In order to look at the issue adequately, it is important to look at controlled studies of SIDS. The studies they examined took one or both of the following approaches: either they looked for an association between DTP immunisation and SIDS, and conducted a cohort study of children vaccinated and not vaccinated; or they conducted a case-control study in which children who died of SIDS were compared with other children, to see whether the SIDS cases were more likely to have received DTP in the interval before they died. Another approach involved comparison of the timing of SIDS deaths in respect of DTP immunisation to see whether SIDS deaths were clustered in the few days following vaccination. The authors state that since only those children who were immunised and who died of SIDS are included in this latter method there is less possibility of detecting an increased risk than in the other approaches.

The Institute of Medicine report concluded that all controlled studies which have compared immunised and non-immunised children had found either no association,[5,6,7] or a decreased risk of cot death among immunised children.[8,9] Out of the four studies[8-11] which looked at the relationship between the timing of immunisation and the occurrence of cot death, only one showed an increased risk.[9] In this study four deaths were reported within 3 days of vaccination compared with the expected 1.38 deaths. These children had been vaccinated at older ages than their controls, which might mean that they had other unrecognised risk factors for cot death unrelated to vaccination.[4]

The committee concluded that there was no evidence to indicate a causal relationship between the diphtheria, tetanus and whooping cough vaccine and cot death.[4] The report also points out that because cot death occurs primarily in the first year of life, when babies are being immunised, some cases following immunisation are to be expected.

Since publication of this report, a large case control study in New Zealand has also shown a decreased risk of cot death among immunised babies compared with non-immunised children.[12]

Scheibner (1993) also suggests that, when Japan altered the routine immunisation schedule to begin at two years of age, cot death was eliminated.[1] She considers this to be evidence that the vaccine causes cot death. In Japan, routine information on cot death is not collected (*personal communication*). The only information available concerns claims made under the vaccination compensation system. When the age of immunisation was raised, claims for cot death associated with immunisation fell to zero.[13] This does not mean that cot death no longer occurred (that information is not available), only that the cases occurring at about the same time as immunisation declined. This is not unexpected, as children were no longer being immunised at the peak age for cot death.

Between 1988 and 1993, the number of deaths attributed to cot death fell dramatically in the UK, New Zealand, Australia, the Netherlands, Norway, Denmark and Ireland.[2] In England and Wales the decline was over 70%. This coincided with a Department of Health campaign which encouraged breastfeeding and advised parents that babies should be put on their backs or sides to sleep; should not be over-wrapped or overheated, and should not be exposed to cigarette smoke.

The drop in the incidence of cot death has also coincided with the diphtheria, tetanus and whooping cough vaccine uptake rate rising from 71% in 1988 to 91% in 1993. There has also been a change in the timing of immunisation, resulting in the primary course being completed when a child is 4 months rather than 11 months old. Since the immunisation schedule was speeded up there has been a small decrease in the percentage of deaths attributed to cot death among babies younger than 6 months old.[14] In countries which give the diphtheria, tetanus and whooping cough vaccine when a child is 6 months old, there is an identical pattern of cot death in 6-month-old children as in the countries where the vaccine is given earlier.[15]

The evidence strongly suggests that there is no relationship between immunisation and Sudden Infant Death Syndrome (cot death).

ASTHMA

Over the past 20 years there has been a real increase in the frequency of asthma among children and adults. Over the same period there has been a rise in both the uptake and the number of vaccines given. Suggested reasons for the increase in asthma include increased pollution and immunisation, but few studies have been specifically designed to investigate a link between asthma and immunisation. Corne (1994) looked at the few studies that have examined the influence of early viral infection on the development of asthma.[16] These studies suggest that, when an infant is exposed to the viral infections of an older brother or sister, this protects the infant against developing an allergy. Corne concluded that:

- vaccination could provoke the same immune response as a viral infection, which has been found to be associated with reduced allergy; or

- by protecting the child against viral infections, vaccination might reduce the protective effect that these infections have on the development of an allergy.

Odent (1994) reported a study (conducted in a number of countries) of the health of children and teenagers who had only been breastfed for the first 6 months of their lives.[17] It was found that, of these children, those who had been given whooping cough vaccine were five times more likely to have been diagnosed as asthmatic than the children who had not been vaccinated. Such differences were not found with diagnoses of other conditions (particularly, eczema). So further research is needed using different methods. This finding raises an important issue, but more detail about Odent's report is needed. In particular, no information was given about how the sample of children was selected. (It is understood that it was a self-selected sample, which introduces the possibility of bias.[18]) And there was no information about how the asthma diagnosis was reported.

Other studies have not found an association between allergies and whooping cough vaccination. Odent's report prompted a group of GPs in Bristol to look at the information for 2146 children in their three practices, but they could find no association between whooping cough immunisation and asthma.[19] In Sweden, a controlled trial of whooping cough vaccine was conducted where 9829 infants were given three doses of either a two-component vaccine, a five-component vaccine, an American whole-cell vaccine, or diphtheria and tetanus vaccine. When the children were about 2½, their parents were asked three standard questions about wheezing, itchy rashes and sneezing. There was no significant difference between the different vaccine groups in the proportions of children with these symptoms. These findings should be taken seriously. This was a large, well-conducted, forward-looking study which sought information about allergy using standard questions. The researchers are planning further in-depth assessment of 720 of the children when they are 7 years old, which will further clarify the issue.[20]

The 1970 Child Health and Education Study (CHES) is based on all children born in England, Scotland and Wales during one week of April 1970. The children and their parents are surveyed at intervals and various aspects of their health, development and education are studied. By 1975 information was available for 80% (13,135) of the original sample. For the first time in a national cohort study the information was analysed to find out if there were any recognisable adverse effects from immunisation. In contrast with Odent's finding, the children in the CHES study who had not been immunised against whooping cough were more likely to have had attacks of wheeziness.[21] In this study, children who did not have the whooping cough vaccine were also more likely to have convulsions or speech defects, to be smaller, to have poor scores on various tests, or to be rated as intellectually abnormal.[22] This finding may also be a reflection of the decision not to immunise a child on the basis of their medical or family history, or because of the change in recommendations over time. (In the past, a personal or family history of allergy was regarded as a reason not to immunise.) Follow-up studies when the children were 10 showed that the children who had completed a primary course of immunisations were a healthy group in comparison with those who were not immunised. They also scored more highly in various educational tests of reading and maths and were less likely to be thin or shorter than average. They were also less likely to have attacks of wheeziness.[23]

OTHER CONDITIONS

Is mass immunisation the cause of autism, AIDS, severe measles infection, multiple sclerosis and immune deficiency problems such as leukaemia?

Harris Coulter, an American researcher and homeopath, has suggested that a range of conditions are due to mass immunisation.[24] These conditions include autism, learning disorders, dyslexia and an increase in violent crime. Coulter based this theory on the observation that these conditions have all increased since mass immunisation began in 1945 and that immunisation can cause inflammation of the brain of varying severity. He notes, for example, that people involved in violent crime have a high incidence of having suffered inflammation of the brain, but he provides no evidence about the causes of this. It has been pointed out that there have been so many changes in society since 1945, including the widespread availability of television, that it is unclear why mass vaccination was deemed to be the cause of various social ills.[25]

Many of these conditions have increased in the population since 1945. However, sometimes this is unlikely to be a true increase but one based on a growing recognition of the conditions. For example, autism was first described in 1944 and the condition became widely accepted very gradually. As the definition of autism has broadened, a rise in the number of cases was to be expected.[25] An association between two events in time does not prove that one causes, or is even linked to, the other (for further discussion on autism see page 40).

Cancer in childhood is a rare condition. The yearly incidence for all types of cancer is about 110 to 130 in every million children. One third of all childhood cancers are leukaemias and, of these, 80% are acute lymphoblastic leukaemia – the most common type of cancer in childhood.[26]

Little is known about the causes of childhood cancer. In two case-control studies immunisation was found to protect against the development of acute lymphoblastic leukaemia, as well as other cancers. Children who had been immunised were significantly less likely to develop cancer than those who had not been immunised.[27,28] The protective effect of immunisation remained after all children under 2 who had been diagnosed with cancer were excluded from the analysis. Ill health caused by the condition could itself be a reason not to immunise.

It has been suggested that there is a connection between vaccination and multiple sclerosis (MS). This has probably arisen because measles antibodies have been found in fluid taken from the spinal cord of patients with MS. It has been suggested that the rise in measles antibody during deteriorating periods of MS points to a link between the virus and the disease process,[29] but this does not mean that measles causes MS. There is no evidence to suggest this process happens after receiving the measles vaccine In fact, researchers in one region of Sweden have already observed a dramatic decrease in MS since the introduction of the measles vaccination. However, they stress that further research is needed before any firm conclusions can be drawn.[30]

AIDS is a complex condition caused by the human immunodeficiency virus (HIV). Over the past 15 years incidences of this condition have increased worldwide. The geographical distribution of AIDS does not correspond with those countries which have high immunisation rates. There is no evidence at all to connect immunisation with AIDS.

ATYPICAL (NON-TYPICAL) MEASLES

In her book, Scheibner (1993) refers to a 'new disease' – atypical measles – which she describes as an 'especially vicious form of measles only affecting vaccinated children and with a high death rate'.[1]

In the 1960s measles vaccines using the killed measles virus were developed. Although these gave protection against measles after two or three doses, their use was discontinued in the late 1960s when up to 15% of those who were vaccinated developed a severe atypical measles infection after being exposed to a wild measles virus.[31] There have also been a few reports of serious atypical measles occurring in children who had previously received a weakened measles vaccine, but the extent of this phenomenon is not known.[32] Atypical measles is a recognised condition identified by a high and prolonged fever, a rash, pneumonia and swelling caused by an excess of fluid in the tissues. It should not be confused with 'mini-measles' (characterised by a mild fever, a general feeling of being unwell and a rash) which is not uncommon in those who have had the live measles vaccine.

DO THE VACCINE VIRUSES LIE DORMANT IN THE BODY AND REACTIVATE LATER, CAUSING MORE SERIOUS DAMAGE?

It is well recognised that following some natural viral infections the virus can become latent and reactivate later. For example, subacute sclerosing panencephalitis (SSPE) is a rare late after-effect of natural measles infection, caused by the measles virus reactivating after a period of latency. Following chickenpox, the virus (varicella zoster) which causes the disease becomes dormant in the cells of the spinal cord. It may reactivate after a period of several decades and cause shingles.[33]

In a study of 290 cases of SSPE registered in England and Wales from 1970 to 1989, 81% had had natural measles infection. The measles vaccine had been given in 20 cases; in 10 cases natural measles was also reported, and it could not be positively excluded in the remainder of the 20 cases. The estimated risk of SSPE after being vaccinated with measles was no greater than 0.14 in 100,000 doses, compared with the rate of SSPE following natural measles infection of 4 in 100,000 cases.[34] The incidence of SSPE has fallen with the reduction in measles resulting from vaccination.[35]

From 1981 in the United States, over 700 healthy children and young people were immunised with the varicella vaccine. There were six reported cases of zoster – a rate of 14 cases per 100,000 person-years. The expected incidence for this age group is 20 to 60 cases per 100,000 person-years so this result is not surprising.[36] Children with leukaemia who have had chickenpox tend to develop zoster at a much higher rate than normal children.[37] However, studies among children with leukaemia who have had the varicella vaccine show that the incidence of zoster following vaccination is lower than after natural infection.[38, 39]

9. The diseases and vaccines

MEASLES

Incidence of measles in England and Wales

Figure 1 (page 13) shows information on the incidence of measles since 1940 when this information started to be collected. Before routine immunisation began in 1968, 90 to 95% of the population had had measles by the age of 10, with the incidence highest in 3- to 5-year-olds.[1] Measles is now rare as a result of high vaccination rates.

Complications of measles virus infection

For most well-nourished, healthy children living in an industrialised country measles is an unpleasant, but not life-threatening, illness. Children with the disease will usually have a rash, a fever, red and painful eyes, a cough and cold. They will usually be off their food, feel miserable, dislike light and feel unwell for about five days. Measles is more likely to lead to severe complications such as pneumonia or encephalitis (inflammation of the brain) and to death in children who have an underlying condition such as difficulty in fighting infections or who are poorly nourished. Children living in developing countries are particularly at risk. However, this does not mean that previously healthy, well-nourished children are not at risk from the complications of measles. Between 1970 and 1983, over half the deaths from measles in this country occurred in previously healthy children, 90% of whom were of an age where they could already have been immunised and protected by the vaccine.[2]

The risk of complications and death from measles is highest in young children and adults. Studies conducted in England and Wales have shown that 1 in 15 children with measles develop complications including pneumonia, middle ear infection and convulsions. About 1 in 100 children with measles have convulsions;[3] 1 in 70 children with measles are admitted to hospital and, from 1980 to 1989, 126 deaths in England and Wales were directly associated with measles.[4] Pneumonia is the most common cause of death associated with measles. Inflammation of the brain is reported at a rate of 1 in 5000 cases of measles.[5] About 15% of patients with inflammation of the brain die and another 25 to 35% have permanent brain damage.[6] A rarer complication of measles, subacute sclerosing panencephalitis (SSPE), is caused by the measles virus reactivating after being dormant. This condition destroys the central nervous system and causes death. In England and Wales between 1970 and 1989, SSPE occurred at a rate of about 4 in 100,000 cases. It presents about seven years after a measles infection. The risk of SSPE is about 18 times higher if a child gets measles in the first year of life than one who has measles after the age of 5.[7]

Measles vaccine

The vaccine's effectiveness in preventing measles

In 1964 a trial began in England and Wales to assess the immediate and long-term protection offered by measles vaccines. Over 36,000 children were given either live measles vaccine (9538 children), vaccine containing the killed virus followed by the live vaccine (10,434 children), or were not vaccinated (16,239 children).[8] The children have been monitored at regular intervals. The most recent monitoring was in 1991, 27 years after the start of the trial.[9]

In the first five years of the trial, live measles vaccine was found to be 91% effective in protecting against measles. After 21 years it was reported that the incidence of measles in the previous nine years was 15 times greater in the unvaccinated group than in the group who had received live vaccine. During the 21-year follow up, more of the cases of measles that occurred in the vaccinated group were described as 'mild' than cases among the unvaccinated group.[8]

Among the group who received vaccine containing the killed virus followed by live vaccine (a system that has not been used in the UK since 1968) no serious atypical measles cases were reported (see page 29).

Length of immunity

The follow-up in 1991 showed that there was still protection from the live measles vaccine given in 1964 and there was no evidence of a decline in the vaccine's effectiveness.[9]

Markowitz *et al.* (1990) reviewed studies to determine the duration and quality of vaccine-induced immunity.[10] As previously mentioned, secondary vaccine failure was found to be uncommon. Several risk factors for this loss of immunity have been identified. These include vaccination at an age when a mother's antibodies might still be present in a child (before the child is one). Markowitz *et al.* consider that there are still many unresolved issues concerning the duration of vaccine-induced immunity and of secondary vaccine failure. For example, in people who have vaccine-induced immunity, their immunity may be boosted by frequent exposure to wild measles, but how this contributes to lifelong immunity is not known.[11] As the disease becomes less common there will be less of this boosting effect and immunity may be reduced.

Adverse reactions following the measles vaccine

Between 1970 and 1980, 10,035 children were vaccinated with measles vaccine and were kept under supervision to check for any symptoms.[12] Three weeks after immunisation a health visitor asked the children's parents for details of any symptoms during the 14 days after the vaccination. Of all the children, 71% (7134) remained well; 20% (2011) had symptoms described as mild, 8% (780) as moderate and 1% (110) as severe.

The symptoms most frequently reported were mild malaise (that is, a general feeling of being unwell) and fever for two to three days. Others included diarrhoea, vomiting, cold, cough and sore eyes. Bronchitis and infection of the middle ear occurred in 0.3% and 0.5%, and a rash in 10%; 5% of the children were seen by their GP and 11 children (0.1%) were admitted to hospital in the 14 days after vaccination. Eleven children (0.1%) had convulsions between the fifth and eleventh day after their vaccination. These children were all monitored through their hospital records and GPs and none of them had further convulsions or problems during the follow-up period, which ranged from one to ten years depending on the year of vaccination. Many of their symptoms could easily have nothing to do with the vaccination.

In a more recent study into adverse effects after the MMR vaccine, vaccination records were linked with hospital admission records. The rate of convulsions attributable to the measles vaccine within 6 to 11 days of the MMR vaccination was found to be even lower than in the earlier study, with a risk of 1 in 3000 doses.[13]

More serious complications such as inflammation of the brain have only rarely been reported following measles immunisation, at a rate of 1 in 1 million doses. As this rate is similar to that of brain inflammation of unknown cause occurring over the same time period in a similar age group, it is difficult to say whether it is actually caused by the vaccine.[14] In a study of 290 cases of SSPE registered in England and Wales between 1970 and 1989, the estimated maximum risk following the measles vaccine was no greater than 0.14 in 100,000 vaccinations. The risk of SSPE was found to be 29 times more likely following a natural attack of measles disease than following measles vaccine.[7]

The risk of serious neurological illness following measles vaccine was also assessed in the National Childhood Encephalopathy (brain disease) Study in England, Scotland and Wales between 1976 and 1979. Of the 16 cases of serious neurological illness which began within 7 to 14 days after measles vaccination, all were normal after one year, except two cases with minor problems.[15]

Table 2 – Severe complications of measles virus infection and risks of live measles vaccine (per 10,000 children)

Complication	Risk after disease	Risk after immunisation
Convulsions	100	3
Inflammation of the brain	2–10	0.01
SSPE	0.4	0.014

Crohn's disease and measles vaccination

Crohn's disease is a disease in which the intestines become swollen, inflamed and ulcerated, causing pain, diarrhoea, weight loss and lack of energy. Symptoms appear in people aged 16 onwards. Factors suggested to be associated with the development of the disease include smoking, living in an urban environment,[16] not having been breastfed,[17] and infections.[18]

Some studies have suggested that measles infection, especially at a young age, or even before birth, may be associated with Crohn's disease.[18-20] Following on from this, a group of researchers in the UK examined the possibility that measles vaccination might also be associated with Crohn's disease. In 1995, they published a study on this topic. In this study, the frequency of Crohn's disease was compared in a group who received measles vaccine in 1964 with that in two historical comparison groups. Although the researchers found an association, they stated that 'it does not show a causal relation'.[21]

In the commentary which accompanied the above publication and subsequent correspondence, the research was criticised for several important reasons. These criticisms included:

- the control groups were not comparable in age, geographical distribution, and other factors which may have influenced the risk of inflammatory bowel disease; and

- the history of Crohn's disease was not gathered in a standard way. It was well documented that the vaccinated group had received measles vaccine and a history of measles disease was also available. They were also specifically asked if they had Crohn's disease. However, in the control groups it was only assumed that they had not been vaccinated against measles and information on Crohn's disease was collected on the basis of answers to a question about their general state of health, rather than to a direct question.[22-27]

Towards the end of 1997, two studies were presented showing no link between Crohn's disease and measles vaccination.[28,29] The weight of evidence is firmly against an association between Crohn's disease and measles vaccination. Studies have also thrown doubt on the supposed link between measles infection and Crohn's disease.[30-34] A recent study showed no connection between measles infection in utero and Crohn's disease.[35] The accompanying editorial[36] reviewed the evidence to date linking measles disease and Crohn's infection and concluded that 'the current evidence does not prove a causal link'. The World Health Organization has also examined all the relevant data and has concluded 'Current scientific evidence does not permit a causal link to be drawn between the measles virus and chronic inflammatory bowel disease.'[37] Since these reviews were published, further work has emerged in which no link between measles virus and inflammatory bowel disease could be demonstrated.[38]

Measles/rubella mass immunisation campaign 1994

In 1994 a mass campaign was mounted to immunise all children between 5 and 16 against measles and rubella. Mumps immunisation was not included as there was no medical evidence for a need. In 1994, a number of sources showed that measles was on the increase, with a high proportion of cases in children aged over 10. Studies of blood serum also suggested that 14% of school children were susceptible to measles. Mathematical calculations predicted that this level of susceptibility was high enough to make a measles epidemic likely. This epidemic would be between 100,000 and 200,000 cases, with up to 50 deaths.[39] An epidemic of measles in Scotland in 1994 illustrated what might occur in England and Wales.[40]

This situation had arisen for several reasons. Firstly, uptake of the measles vaccine before the introduction of MMR in 1988 was poor. Fewer than 60% of 2-year-olds were vaccinated, and these children were now in school. Secondly, about 10% of vaccinated children would not have responded to the vaccine. Also the decrease in measles over the previous five years meant that the opportunity for unprotected children to get immunity through natural infection had greatly reduced.

This has proved to be an extremely successful strategy in preventing the spread of measles infection. There were only 148 cases of confirmed measles in the 18 months from January 1995 to June 1996. Not one of these confirmed cases has occurred in children vaccinated in the campaign.[41]

Adverse reactions to the measles and rubella vaccine

During the measles/rubella campaign, over 7 million children aged 5 to 16 received the vaccine. The campaign received considerable publicity and raised awareness of both the dangers of measles and the potential for side effects after vaccination.[42]

The estimated rate at which adverse reactions were reported was 1 in every 6700 children immunised. Most reactions were minor. Some 530 children (0.007%) had a serious reaction, but none of these children died. There were 91 reports of serious neurological reactions. Of these, 11 children (1 in 730,000) were reported with encephalitis (inflammation of the brain), and a definite diagnosis was made in just six of these children. None of the children had the vaccine identified as the cause for inflammation of the brain and 10 of the children recovered completely. The remaining child suffered paralysis but had no change in his antibody levels. This suggests that he was already immune and it was unlikely that his condition had been caused by the vaccine. The number of reports of this condition was less than the number expected to occur if there had been no vaccination campaign.

One child with SSPE developed symptoms one month after being immunised. The usual incubation period for SSPE is much longer (an average of seven years) and in this case the child was exposed to a wild measles infection some years earlier. So it is unlikely that the vaccine was responsible. There were three reports of Guillain-Barré syndrome – one of the affected children had a chest infection at the time of immunisation, and a second child had a rare form of Guillain-Barré syndrome. There were not enough details on the third case. Considering the known pattern of cases of Guillain-Barré syndrome, between one and seven cases would be expected to occur each month in the population, regardless of immunisation. So the number of reported cases matches the usual frequency of the disease.[43] Other work has shown that there is no link between measles vaccination and the Guillain-Barré syndrome.[44]

Serious adverse reactions were rare and, where there was a clear link between the reaction and the vaccine, all the children made a complete recovery. For children who did not make a recovery, there was no conclusive evidence to support any association with the vaccine. These reactions must be considered in light of the likely consequences of a large epidemic of measles. The long-term serious effects of measles are much greater than those potentially associated with vaccination. It is impossible to prove that an epidemic would have occurred in 1995 without just letting one happen but, mathematical models, together with observations of trends, provided the strongest possible prediction that an epidemic was going to occur. The only alternative course of action would have been to do nothing but, in the face of the evidence, 'it would have been indefensible not to intervene'.[45]

Future policy

No country has succeeded in eliminating measles without a second dose of vaccine. A single dose of MMR vaccine gives protection against measles and mumps in around 90% of people and protects about 95% of people against rubella. So, if 92% of children are given MMR vaccine, with measles vaccine being protective in 90% of people, only 83% of each year's birth group are protected. Over time, the number of unprotected children builds up and every few years reaches a level which allows an epidemic of measles to occur.

From October 1996, all children except those with a valid medical reason, should receive two doses of MMR vaccine. The Department of Health recommends that the first is given shortly after the first birthday and the second dose before starting school.[46]

MUMPS

Complications of mumps infection

Before the immunisation programme was introduced epidemics of mumps occurred every three years in England and Wales. It was the commonest cause of viral meningitis in children, affecting about 1 in 400 children. Other complications include deafness, inflammation of the ovaries or testes (which rarely leads to sterility), and inflammation of the pancreas.[47] These occur more often in adults than in children, with inflammation of the testicles affecting as many as 38% of teenage boys and men who suffer the illness.[48]

Mumps vaccine

The mumps vaccine was introduced into this country in 1988, in combination with the measles and rubella vaccine, for 1-year-old children. Owing to the increased risk of complications of the disease in adults, it is particularly important that as many children as possible are vaccinated to prevent adults catching mumps.

The live mumps vaccine is prepared in a cell culture made from chick embryos. More than 90% of people who are susceptible to mumps develop antibodies after a single dose. In vaccinated populations, monitoring over a period of at least 25 years has shown immunity to be long lasting.[49]

Adverse reactions to mumps vaccine

Reactions to the mumps part of MMR vaccine are generally mild, with mini-mumps occurring in about 1% of children three weeks after the vaccine. More serious reactions, such as meningitis, occur less frequently.

To assess the risk of aseptic meningitis in the UK, during 1990 and 1991 paediatricians were asked to report all confirmed and suspected cases of meningoencephalitis occurring in children under 16 within six weeks of MMR vaccine to the British Paediatric Surveillance Unit. The risk based on confirmed cases was estimated to be very low at four out of every million children vaccinated. All cases of meningitis occurred in those who received a vaccine containing a specific strain of the virus 'Urabe'. However, information from one district suggested a much higher risk of about 1 in 4000 doses. To assess the true risk a study was set up in 13 districts linking vaccination records with hospital records. The true risk was estimated to be about 1 in 11,000 doses and all cases were linked to the vaccine containing the 'Urabe' strain of the mumps virus; this is no longer used in this country.[50] Since changing the vaccines from the Urabe type, there has been no single meningitis case associated with mumps vaccine and around 2 million doses have been used.

Impact of mumps vaccine

Within two years of the vaccine being introduced, there was a dramatic and rapid decline in the number of cases of mumps, shown by GP reports and laboratory reports.

RUBELLA (GERMAN MEASLES)

Rubella (German measles) is a mild disease with few complications, unless caught in early pregnancy. The disease is often confused with other viral illnesses and a history of rubella disease alone may not be enough to be certain that a person is actually immune.

The link between rubella in pregnancy and birth defects was first recognised by an Australian eye specialist, Gregg, in 1941. He noticed an unusually large number of infants with cataracts and further investigation revealed that their mothers had had rubella infections in pregnancy during the Australian outbreak of 1940. Similar reports followed from Australia, Sweden, the United States and the UK and the role of rubella in congenital cataracts was confirmed. The coincidence of heart disease and deafness was also noted.[51] A major rubella epidemic in the USA in 1964–65 resulted in around 20,000 rubella-damaged babies and this highlighted the need to prevent this infection.

Before GPs had to start reporting cases of rubella (1988), the main sources of information were the Royal College of General Practitioners reporting scheme and laboratory reports. The National Congenital Rubella Surveillance Programme set up in 1971 showed an epidemic cycle every 3 to 5 years.

Complications of rubella and congenital rubella syndrome

Joint pain and arthritis are frequent complications of rubella in adults, especially in women.[52] Thrombocytopenia (a reduction in the number of platelets in the blood) occurs in 1 in 4000 cases of natural rubella.[53]

If a woman gets rubella early in her pregnancy it can result in congenital rubella syndrome in the baby. Miller E *et al.* (1982)[54] showed that, when rubella was caught during pregnancy, 80% of babies became infected when the mother was infected in the first 12 weeks, 67% during weeks 13 and 14, with a steady decline to 25% at the end of 26 weeks. In babies that became infected, rubella-associated defects occurred in 100% of pregnancies infected in the first 11 weeks, 50% of those from 11 to 12 weeks and 35% of those from 13 to 16 weeks. The most common permanent defects are deafness, learning difficulties, cataracts, heart defects, sight problems and cerebral palsy. Diabetes has also been observed in adolescents and young adults who became infected before birth.[52]

Rubella vaccine

The live rubella virus currently used in the UK for vaccine is the 'RA 27/3' strain. This is grown in human cell cultures. One dose of the vaccine gives long-term immunity in more than 95% of cases. However, there have been reports of people who were previously shown to be immune to rubella, whether following immunisation or disease, who have lost this protection. Women who are planning a pregnancy should be screened to make sure that they are immune.

Adverse effects of rubella vaccine

Reactions such as a fever, a sore throat, enlarged glands, a rash, arthritis and joint pain may occur following immunisation. Symptoms usually begin one to three weeks after receiving the vaccine and are usually mild and temporary. The estimated incidence of acute arthritis is 13 to 15%, mostly in adult women. The pains may last only a few days, or may recur with lessening severity and with longer intervals between episodes.[52] However, the 1991 Institute of Medicine Report of adverse effects following rubella vaccine could not find any reliable estimates of there being an excess risk of chronic arthritis following vaccination against rubella.[55] The report suggested further research was needed. Two recent studies have failed to confirm an increased risk of joint problems after rubella vaccine.[56, 57] A Canadian study[58] showed 'only marginally significant differences in persistent or recurrent joint manifestations between rubella vaccine and placebo reactions'.

Farrington *et al.* (1995) found there to be a risk of thrombocytopenia in 1 out of every 29,000 vaccinated.[13] This is about one eighth of the risk after suffering from the disease. A French review reported a lower rate. The course of the condition was similar to acute thrombocytopenia not associated with vaccination and 90% of children made a complete recovery.[59]

Rubella vaccination in pregnancy

Rubella vaccine should not be given to pregnant women and women should avoid getting pregnant for one month after being vaccinated, as there is, in theory, a risk to the fetus for the first few weeks. However, pregnant women have sometimes been immunised, or become pregnant sooner than the recommended interval. Follow-up of such cases has shown that, of the 123 births reported to the National Congenital Rubella Surveillance Programme between 1980 and 1995, no child was born with defects which could be linked to congenital rubella infection (*personal communication* – P. Tookey, NCRSP). The maximum theoretical risk of fetal damage following rubella vaccination in pregnancy or within three months of conception has been calculated using information combined from the USA, Sweden, Germany and the UK. The observed risk of congenital rubella syndrome is zero and the maximum theoretical risk in an infant whose mother's pregnancy is complicated by rubella vaccination is very low at less than 0.75%.[60] Continued follow-up of such women is important to assess the effect of vaccination in pregnancy.

Rubella vaccination policy and its effect on rubella

Rubella vaccination was introduced into this country in 1970 for school girls and susceptible adult women. This selective immunisation strategy was chosen to provide protection against rubella in pregnancy rather than to eliminate the disease from the country. MMR immunisation was introduced in 1988 for all one-year-old children. The aim of this policy was to eliminate rubella from the community and break the chain of the disease being passed from children to pregnant women. The policy was changed because surveys showed that, despite the high vaccine uptake in girls and adult women, 2 to 3% of adult women were likely to remain susceptible. So, in order to eliminate rubella-related defects, it was necessary to interrupt the circulation of the wild rubella virus.[61]

Uptake of the MMR vaccine has been high and there has been a reduction in the number of cases in children under 5 and among pregnant women, fewer abortions because of rubella disease or contact with rubella, and fewer children born with rubella-related defects. The risk of susceptible women contracting rubella from young children has been substantially reduced since the MMR vaccine was introduced.

In 1993 there were local outbreaks of rubella infection, largely affecting young males.[62] This group of males had never been included in a rubella vaccination programme and the outbreaks may be a reflection of delayed exposure to rubella infection because of high MMR coverage.

Following the 1994 measles and rubella immunisation campaign for children aged 5 to 16, rubella immunisation of school girls was stopped. This was because MMR vaccination rates in children under 2 are high, and girls between the ages of 5 and 16 who did not receive the vaccine will have had the opportunity to have the measles and rubella vaccine, thus covering any gaps in immunity. However, when children have their school-leaving immunisations, any boys and girls who have not had the measles and rubella vaccine should be offered the MMR vaccine. Single rubella antigen is also recommended for susceptible women who are planning pregnancy and for non-immune women after giving birth. It will be important to continue to monitor trends in rubella infection. The full impact of the campaign on the risk of congenital rubella is likely to become apparent in five to ten years' time.[41]

MMR VACCINE

Combination vaccines, in which a number of antigens are given together, are a good idea because they mean that a child needs fewer injections but at the same time is protected against more than one disease. The cost of vaccination is also reduced. However, safety and effectiveness remain the most important considerations and research must show that the combined vaccine is as effective as single ones and that side effects are not increased.

Considerable experience with MMR vaccine in many countries has shown it to be safe and very effective. In the US there has been over 25 years' experience of the vaccine with hundreds of millions of doses of vaccine given. The many studies reviewed by Markowitz and Katz [63] show that the combined vaccine gives the same high rates of seroconversion and that the risk of reactions in people susceptible to all three antigens does not increase.

A combined measles, mumps and rubella vaccine was introduced into this country in 1988 for children aged 1 to 2 years. The aim was to eliminate measles, mumps, rubella and congenital rubella syndrome. It was introduced only after high enough levels of measles vaccine had been achieved to suggest that the MMR coverage rate would be enough to stop the spread of the viruses. It has been well accepted, with over 90% of children receiving the vaccine by the time they are two.[64] Success rates of 90 to 95% for the measles component, 90 to 95% for mumps and 97 to 99% for rubella are found.[65] The viruses cannot be passed on from a recently immunised child.

The adverse effects of MMR vaccine are the same as for the individual components. (For further details see the individual sections on mumps, measles and rubella.)

Autism

Recently a number of parents have become concerned that their children have developed autism following the MMR vaccine. Autism is a disorder in which there is an abnormality of social interaction and language and obsessional tendencies. It was first described by Kanner in 1943, many years before MMR vaccine was developed.[66] There is a broad range of severity and many children without classical autism may be labelled as having behaviour which falls within the 'autistic spectrum'. The diagnosis is usually made in the second year of life but international classifications allow for the diagnosis to made in anyone with the appropriate features presenting before 36 months old.[67] It is therefore inevitable that in some children the timing of diagnosis will be in close proximity to the receipt of the MMR vaccine. This does not prove a causal connection. Many conditions may give rise to autism[68] and there may be a genetic element in most cases.[69,70] Autism is among the recognised abnormalities affecting children with the congenital rubella syndrome.[71] There is some evidence that postnatal encephalitis may in some cases result in children developing autism, however this is not proven and it would only explain a small proportion of cases.[72] There is no evidence to suggest that viral infections may give rise to autism without there being an encephalitic illness severe enough to require hospital admission.

It has been suggested that there has been an increase in children with autism but it is unclear whether there has been a true increase or perhaps a better awareness of the condition and its wide spectrum.[73] In summary there is little biological plausibility in a link between MMR vaccine and autism and no studies to demonstrate such a link. To investigate such a link would require a well designed epidemiological study.

In February 1998, Wakefield and his colleagues published a paper in *The Lancet* in which they described the case histories of 12 children.[74] These children were reported to have developed behavioural symptoms such as loss of developmental milestones including loss of language, in addition to intestinal symptoms: diarrhoea, pain and bloating. Nine of the children were subsequently diagnosed as having autism or an autistic spectrum disorder and the three remaining children to have either encephalitis (one following vaccination, one following a viral illness) or a disintegrative disorder. Their bowel symptoms were diagnosed as colitis (inflammation of the bowel) and hyperplasia (increased production of normal cells). In eight of these children the symptoms were linked by their parents and/or doctors to MMR vaccination. In two no such link was made; in one child the symptoms followed natural measles infection and in another, followed ear infections.

The authors suggest a mechanism for this syndrome: intestinal symptoms leading to over-absorption from the diet of certain protein parts (peptides). These peptides may have direct or indirect effects which result in a disruption of brain development. Intestinal problems have been reported previously in children with autistic spectrum disorders, but the combination of symptoms may also have occurred by chance. Wakefield *et al.* acknowledge that this is a highly selected group of children, referred to them because of their previous work looking at a possible link between inflammatory bowel disease and measles vaccination.[21] This means that these findings are not representative of the whole MMR vaccinated child population. They also state that virus studies have not been completed on these children and no association between MMR and the syndrome was proven. Indeed, a valid investigation of such an association would require a study involving very large numbers of vaccinated as well as unvaccinated children, in which the incidence of the syndrome was compared between the two groups.

In a commentary published in the same edition of *The Lancet*, Chen and DeStefano[75] emphasise that since the mid-1960s, measles vaccine has been given to hundreds of millions of people worldwide and MMR vaccine to tens of millions without them developing either chronic bowel or behavioural problems, and that if MMR does cause such a syndrome it is extremely rare. They consider the paper has serious weaknesses that undermine the authors' suggestion that MMR vaccine may have played a part in the syndrome. They also have doubts about the validity of the suggested mechanism for this syndrome, since in almost all the cases described, the behavioural changes appeared first and parents were less clear about the timing of the onset of abdominal symptoms. Further, there is now a considerable body of research which has failed to confirm a link between IBD and measles (or MMR).

The Wakefield paper concluded, 'We have identified a chronic enterocolitis in children that may be related to neuropsychiatric dysfunction. In most cases, onset of symptoms was after measles, mumps and rubella immunisation. Further investigations are needed to examine this syndrome and its possible relation to the vaccine.' The paper received widespread media coverage and, in spite of the lack of evidence, Dr Wakefield in his public statements advised that the combined MMR vaccine should be withdrawn and the components used separately. On the other hand, another member of the team, a paediatrician, strongly advocated the continuation of the use of the combined vaccine and pointed out how tragic it would be if people stopped being immunised and measles disease became common again.

The data have been looked at very carefully by the Joint Committee on Vaccination and Immunisation (comprising independent scientific experts) which advises the Department of Health. The committee does not feel that this paper provides any reason to change the current immunisation policy.

HAEMOPHILUS INFLUENZAE TYPE B (HIB)

The Hib organism was first isolated and described in 1892. At the time it was thought to be the cause of flu, hence its name. But this theory was later shown not to be true. At any one time, between 1 to 5% of the population carry strains of Hib as a harmless organism. The rate was highest in children under five.[76] Most people become immune in the first few years of life without ever having developed the Hib disease.

Very young babies are protected in the womb by antibodies passed from their mothers, mainly after 32 weeks of pregnancy. They may also be protected, to a lesser extent, by breastfeeding.[76] These antibodies decline after the first few months of life, so children aged 3 months onwards are most at risk of Hib disease until they have built up their own immunity. Invasive Hib disease manifests itself as meningitis, a blockage of the throat (epiglottitis), pneumonia, septic arthritis and cellulitis. Hib meningitis in particular is associated with a high rate of complications. In a study of children who suffered Hib meningitis in their first year and were followed up at 5 years of age, 4% of the children had died in the acute stage of the illness and 8% were found to have significant after-effects including hearing loss, learning difficulties, and cerebral palsy.[77] Before the vaccine was introduced, there were around 1600 infections each year in this country with 60 deaths. One in 600 children had had the disease by the age of 5, and 1 in 800 children developed meningitis.[78]

Invasive Hib infection occurs worldwide, but attack rates vary a great deal and depend on different environmental and genetic factors. Several risk factors for Hib disease have been identified. Most at risk are young children who lack antibodies and those with defects in immunity. Ethnic group has also been found to be important. For example, Aborigines, native American Indians and Alaskan Eskimos have some of the highest attack rates in the world, four to 20 times that of other groups. Although social conditions such as overcrowding, which may increase exposure to infection, may play a part, there must be other reasons for such greatly increased risks. Studies from the USA have also shown that attendance at day care nurseries is associated with a substantially increased risk (two to five times greater) of Hib infection, with the youngest children at greatest risk.[76]

It has been claimed that the widespread introduction of diphtheria, tetanus and whooping cough immunisation has caused an increase in Hib infections.[79,80] However, this can be seen as another example of an association between two events where there is no conclusive evidence of cause and effect.

Hib vaccine

The first vaccine developed against Hib consisted of a purified part of the organism. A major trial in Finland involving over 98,000 children showed that the vaccine was effective in preventing Hib disease in children over 18 months old, but gave no protection to children under 18 months old (those at greatest risk of disease). There were several reports of episodes of Hib disease occurring within one week of vaccination. The significance of these findings has been debated. As the vaccine was not expected to bring about protective immunity until at least a week after immunisation, the occurrence of disease soon after immunisation may be no greater than expected, given the amount of vaccine administered and the natural incidence of disease.[81] These early vaccines were not widely incorporated into immunisation schedules. Further vaccine development showed that, by joining or fusing (conjugating) the purified part of the organism to a carrier protein such as diphtheria toxoid, there was a great improvement in the vaccine's ability to protect against disease, especially in very young children.

Extensive evaluation of four such conjugate vaccines showed that they are well accepted and that serious adverse reactions do not occur. Each has been licensed for use in many countries including the USA, the UK, Finland, Iceland and Germany. High levels of protection (90 to 100%) have been demonstrated.

A large Hib vaccine trial began in the Oxford region in 1991. The Hib vaccine was introduced into four districts, with four others acting as controls. A surveillance system had been set up several years earlier to detect any cases of disease. More than 27,000 children were immunised in the trial, with no cases of disease among infants who were given three doses of vaccine and 11 cases among the control population. This represents a vaccine success rate of 100%. By the end of 1993 there was only one vaccine failure.[82]

When Hib was first introduced a number of vaccines were available from different manufacturers. However, until the evidence became available that it was safe and effective to switch different vaccines within one course, it was advised not to do so. A trial has now shown that administering the improved vaccines in a number of different sequences did not affect the number of infants gaining protection after they were vaccinated, nor did it increase the rate of adverse reactions.[83] On this basis, the Department of Health (1996) has now altered its recommendations.[46] Similarly, there is now enough evidence to show that Hib vaccine and DTP vaccine can be mixed together in particular combinations and given at the same time without weakening their efficiency or increasing the rate of adverse reactions.[84]

Adverse reactions to Hib vaccine

There is now extensive experience of conjugate Hib vaccines used in several countries. By early 1992 it was estimated that 20 million doses had been distributed worldwide. Redness and swelling may occur in 10 to 15% of vaccinated children, more commonly after the first injection. Rates of irritability and fever do not differ significantly in children given the Hib vaccine at the same time as DTP compared with those given DTP alone.[85] Serious reactions due to Hib vaccine have not been reported.

Since the improved Hib vaccine was introduced in 1992, a study of invasive disease occurring in vaccinated infants has been underway to check for vaccine failures. Paediatricians and microbiologists are asked to report all cases of disease in children who had received one or more doses of the Hib vaccine. In the first two years of the study, 26 cases of vaccine failure were identified. Ten children had medical conditions which may have been associated with a reduced response to immunisation. From this, the effectiveness of the vaccine is estimated to be 98%.[86]

Reduction in Hib disease

In every country that has introduced Hib vaccination programmes, there has been a dramatic decline in the incidence of the disease in all age groups, not just those receiving the vaccine. This shows that the vaccine has stopped the Hib bacteria being spread to unvaccinated children. In the first five years of the Hib

Figure 3 Laboratory reports to CDSC (bacteraemia and meningitis) of Haemophilus influenzae, *England and Wales 1989–94*

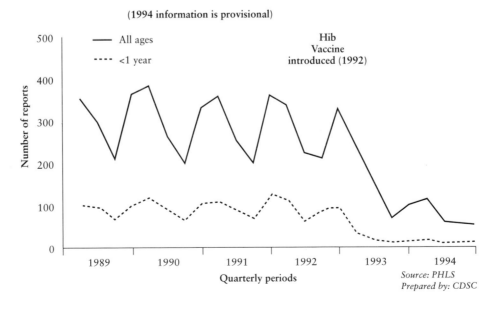

(1994 information is provisional)

Source: PHLS
Prepared by: CDSC

vaccination programme in Finland, the number of cases of Hib meningitis in children aged 0 to 4 fell from 30 in 1986 to zero in 1991.[87] In the USA, information from an intensive laboratory-based active surveillance system and the National Bacterial Meningitis Reporting System were separately evaluated and showed that Hib meningitis decreased by 85% between 1985 and 1991. Increases in doses of Hib vaccine distributed in the USA coincided with steep drops in Hib disease.[88] In the UK between 1992 and 1993 there was an 80% decline in confirmed cases of Hib meningitis and septicaemia (blood poisoning) in children under one,[89] and in 1995 the decline was 95%. Figure 3 shows the marked decline in laboratory reports of Hib infection in all age groups since the vaccine was introduced.

WHOOPING COUGH (PERTUSSIS)

Whooping cough is particularly serious in very young children as they are most at risk of severe complications and death. Whooping cough is also more difficult to diagnose in young children who may not demonstrate the classic 'whoop'.[90] Of the 50 deaths between 1980 and 1991 in England and Wales associated with whooping cough, 28 (56%) occurred in children under 5 months old.[91] In epidemics, death from whooping cough appears to be even more common than reports suggest. During the whooping cough epidemics of the late 1970s and early 1980s, Cherry (1993) found that out of every ten deaths probably caused by whooping cough, only one was actually attributed to the infection.[92] Complications of whooping cough described in a study among 2295 cases in Wales included acute bronchitis (9.8%), temporarily stopping breathing (1.1%), convulsions (0.6%), and two children who had inflammation of the brain.[93] Whooping cough is significantly associated with brain disease in approximately 1 in 10,000 cases.[94]

In older children, the main problem with whooping cough is that it lasts a long time. Since it is also likely that more than one family member will be affected at any one time, it can have a major effect on the family. Many parents who have nursed a child with whooping cough have described changes in the child's behaviour including exhaustion, loss of appetite, disturbed sleeping habits and delays in development. As a result, they may fear for the health and life of their child and experience long periods of lack of sleep themselves.[95]

In a population study of 658 children, the factors that influence the clinical picture of whooping cough and its ability to infect were examined.[96] The disease was found to be lengthy, lasting an average of 50 days, although there were relatively few major complications. The effect of whooping cough immunisation was to lower the spread of the disease within the family. When exposed to whooping cough within the family, about two out of ten immunised children developed the disease, compared with seven out of ten non-immunised children.

From 1977 to 1992, 500 successive cases of confirmed whooping cough were studied in a general practice. Most cases of whooping cough were relatively mild, although there were five cases of pneumonia, one in a critically ill five-week-old baby. Since half the patients did not 'whoop', this could have resulted in underdiagnosis. The disease was most common in 3-year-olds, with a small peak in adults in their 30s, reflecting the age of the parents of children with whooping cough. Six of the adults with whooping cough had a childhood history of the disease. Female and unimmunised patients suffered more severely than others. This survey confirmed previous studies which have demonstrated that whooping cough is under-notified, (the actual incidence was six times greater than the national notification rate during the same period). The author emphasised the importance of high immunisation coverage as the only means of reducing damage and deaths in those too young to be immunised themselves.[97]

Likelihood of an unimmunised child catching the disease

In the only research of its type, it was calculated that a child who had not completed a full course of whooping cough vaccination had a 1 in 6 chance of contracting the disease before his or her tenth birthday.[98] Information from Italy, where uptake of whooping cough vaccine is poor, shows that 25% of children have experienced whooping cough by their fifth birthday.[99]

Whooping cough vaccine

The whooping cough vaccine that is currently used in the UK was developed in the 1940s. It contains at least six active components. A full course of vaccine provides protection against whooping cough in over 80% of people.[100] Many studies have shown that, even when whooping cough immunisation does not provide complete protection against disease, the disease is less severe.[96, 101-103]

Adverse reactions to whooping cough vaccine

This is probably the area of immunisation that causes most concern for parents. The whooping cough vaccine has received more attention than any other, with numerous studies undertaken and papers, comments and letters written both in medical and non-medical publications.

Minor reactions following the diphtheria, tetanus and whooping cough vaccine (known as DTP) are common, with up to 70% of those vaccinated experiencing fever and irritability. It has been observed that children given DTP vaccine have a slightly higher rate of irritability and fever than children given diphtheria and tetanus vaccine.[14]

Convulsions after DTP immunisation are also relatively common, with estimates varying between approximately 1 in 1750 to 1 in 13,400 immunisations. These are usually feverish convulsions and there is no evidence that they injure the central nervous system, represent the onset of epilepsy, or worsen existing diseases of the nervous system. Although there is an increased risk of fits in a child with a personal or family history of convulsions, there is no evidence of an increased risk of other problems of the nervous system developing after immunisation.[104]

In a study in which vaccination records were linked with hospital records, the risk of convulsions up to three days after DTP immunisation was 1 in 12,500 doses and was limited to the third dose. The study covered the period during which the speeded-up schedule was introduced. The authors suggested that this change to the new schedule (2, 3 and 4 months) may have led to a four-fold decrease in feverish convulsions as a result of the DTP vaccine, and so the risk with the new regime is even lower than before.[13]

Baxter (1994) reported on 1500 children seen in an immunisation advisory clinic.[105] These were children with possible medical reasons for not receiving the whooping cough vaccine, or whose parents were unsure whether to have their children vaccinated. Of these, 451 children had histories of problems of the nervous system, 29 were judged to be immune (on the basis of previous history and blood testing) and so were not vaccinated, and the parents of a further 90 children refused to have their child immunised. Some 332 children were immunised with whooping cough vaccine and 2 serious adverse reactions occurred. One was a severe local reaction in a child whose parents had a history of epilepsy and the other was a child who had had multiple abnormalities from birth, who had an infection at the same time and suffered seizures. The family history of the first child was not relevant to the reaction, and the seizures in the second child were likely to be a coincidence, rather than caused by the immunisation. This highlights the importance of weighing up the probability of having whooping cough, plus its risks and complications, against the effectiveness of the vaccine and its possible adverse reactions. For virtually all children, the balance favours vaccination.[106]

The controversy surrounding whooping cough vaccine took hold in 1974. Some doctors at Great Ormond Street Hospital published a paper in which it was suggested that there was a relationship between whooping cough immunisation and serious conditions of the nervous system, in particular epilepsy and learning disorders.[107] This led to a dramatic fall in the uptake of whooping cough vaccine and a rise in cases of whooping cough, with about 100,000 extra cases between 1977 and 1980. It has been suggested that the high awareness of whooping cough during this period was partly due to an increase in the proportion of cases reported. A study in 1980 compared the rates of notifications in three whooping cough outbreaks with those for cases reported to the Royal College of General Practitioners.[108] These reports are made weekly by GPs in selected practices, who have a continuing commitment to report each case diagnosed. As such, they are probably less likely to be influenced by publicity and more likely to provide a true picture of changes in incidence. While there was a four-fold increase in the number of cases of whooping cough reported in 1977–79 compared with the previous outbreak in 1973–75, the Royal College of General Practitioners scheme reports in 1977–79 were twice the number reported in 1973–75. This does suggest that there was an increase in the proportion of cases reported, but still represents a substantial increase in the incidence of whooping cough associated with the decline in the number of children being vaccinated against whooping cough.

Following the events in the mid 1970s experts were commissioned and a major study, known as the National Childhood Encephalopathy Study (NCES), was set up. The study looked at children aged 2 months to 36 months who were admitted to hospital over a three-year period with serious acute illness of the nervous system. For each child studied, two control children were also studied. Many factors were investigated including immunisation histories. The results were published in 1981. On the basis of the information collected, it was concluded that the risk of a previously normal child developing a serious acute illness of the nervous system due to whooping cough immunisation was 1 in 110,000 immunisations, and the risk of suffering permanent brain damage was 1 in 310,000.[15] On this basis, it has been calculated that a GP or health visitor would see one severe reaction in 1500 years.[109]

Since then, further studies and other events have occurred that tend to suggest the risk may be even lower than suggested in the NCES. In 1988 a court case alleged that a child had been brain damaged as a result of receiving the whooping cough vaccine. The judge reviewed all the literature and concluded that he was not convinced beyond reasonable doubt that the vaccine had caused permanent brain damage. The judge stated that he could not totally exclude the possibility but said that, if such problems did occur, they must happen very rarely indeed.[110] It is important to note that, during the course of the study, more than one million doses of vaccine had been administered and no child in the NCES whose nervous system was previously normal suffered permanent brain damage when the onset of the condition was within 48 hours of the vaccine being given.

Three studies conducted in the UK and the USA, accounting for more than 500,000 doses of vaccine, found no cases of encephalopathy.[14,111,112] A large case-control study published in 1994, which included 218,000 children, found no association between the onset of serious illness of the nervous system and the DTP vaccine being given within the previous seven days.[113]

In the USA, the Institute of Medicine set up a committee to conduct a review of literature dealing with the adverse effects of whooping cough and rubella vaccines.[54] The committee spent nearly two years reviewing a wide range of information sources, including case studies, case reports, published and unpublished epidemiological studies, studies in animals and other laboratory studies. When considering disorders of the nervous system and the DTP vaccine (the committee did not separate out whooping cough vaccine from diphtheria and tetanus), they came to the following conclusions.

- **There was insufficient evidence to indicate a causal relation** to aseptic meningitis, chronic damage of the nervous system, Guillain-Barré syndrome, learning disabilities and peripheral mono neuropathy, haemolytic anaemia, juvenile diabetes, attention deficit disorder or thrombocytopenia.

- **The evidence favoured rejection of a causal relation** to infantile spasms, hypsarrhythmias, Reye's syndrome or cot death.

In 1993 in Eire, Kenneth Best was awarded £2.75 million in damages from a vaccine manufacturer. It was judged that he was damaged after receiving whooping cough vaccine from a particular batch which had failed a safety test and so should not have been released. It is important to emphasise that this judgment was not that the vaccine causes problems of the nervous system, but that particular batches of it should never have been released.

The risks to the nervous system have been analysed and re-analysed by seven major committees and they have found no evidence to support the opinion that whooping cough vaccine causes brain damage.[91] The evidence suggests that serious reactions to the vaccine are rare and no long-term adverse reactions have been proven. The benefits of the whooping cough vaccine far outweigh any risks.[114]

Acellular whooping cough vaccines

Research has been in hand for many years to try to produce a vaccine that is at least as effective as the traditional one, but has fewer side effects. There are at least 13 potential vaccines. A trial in Sweden showed that a particular two-component vaccine caused far fewer minor side effects (such as fever, sore arms, fretfulness and so on) than the conventional vaccine.[115] The levels of antibodies produced by the vaccine were also high. Similar findings have resulted from many trials using different acellular vaccines, including one in the UK.[116]

However, it is not always possible to equate antibody levels with protection from a vaccine. The only way to prove that the vaccine is effective is to use it and see if it protects. Since whooping cough has become less common in this country this is not easy to do. Some studies have looked at whether immunisation protects children from catching the disease from their brother or sister. One such study in Japan[117] showed that 84.2% of unimmunised children with brothers or sisters developed whooping cough, whereas only 7.7% or 5.5% developed the disease when they had received either the whole-cell or acellular vaccine respectively. Other family studies suggest that the vaccines are highly effective, but more research is necessary.

Whooping cough is still common in Italy, Germany and Sweden, and a number of large-scale vaccine trials have just been completed in these countries. In the Swedish and Italian trials many different acellular vaccines containing either two, three or five whooping cough components were compared with a standard whole-cell vaccine used in the USA (but not in the UK). The effectiveness of the acellular vaccines was 85% for the five-component vaccine, 84% for each of the three-component vaccines and 59% for the two-component vaccines. The American whole-cell vaccine performed poorly (35% in the Swedish trial and 48% in the Italian trial) but, in the USA, a fourth dose is given routinely in the second year of life and this booster was not included in either of the trials. All the acellular vaccines included in the trials were associated with significantly fewer and milder adverse reactions than the whole-cell vaccine.[118,119]

The whole-cell vaccine used in the UK was part of a Swedish trial between 1993 and 1996 and was found to be highly effective against both mild and severe disease. In Japan, a number of the new vaccines are licensed for use. A trial in the UK showed that whereas the acellular vaccine had fewer side effects than the conventional vaccine in older children, there was little difference when it was given at the UK standard ages of 2, 3 and 4 months.[120] At the end of 1996, a combined diphtheria, tetanus and acellular whooping cough vaccine was licensed for all five doses of DTP given to Japanese children aged from 6 weeks to 6 years.[121] Some other countries have followed suit.

One acellular vaccine is already available in the UK for children who have received diphtheria and tetanus alone as the primary course, and so need the whooping cough vaccine later. As there is little difference in adverse reactions in young infants and the conventional vaccines are slightly more effective than the acellular vaccines, it is unlikely there will be any change in the primary vaccination schedule. There is evidence that whooping cough is commoner in adults than previously recognised.[122,123] For this reason the acellular vaccine might be introduced as preschool and school leavers' boosters. At these ages, whole-cell vaccine is thought to be associated with a high frequency of side effects.

POLIOMYELITIS (POLIO)

Polio is an acute viral infection of the intestines. In a small proportion of cases the infection may extend to the central nervous system, resulting in paralysis. It is common for the infection to go unnoticed. The ratio of undetected to paralysing infection may be 1000 to 1 in children or 75 to 1 in adults.[45]

Polio vaccines

Two types of polio vaccine are available. In this country the live oral polio vaccine has been routinely given since 1962 and the wild polio virus has been eliminated since 1984.[125] Other countries (most of Scandinavia, France, the Netherlands and Finland) use either inactivated (killed) polio vaccine alone, or in combination with the live oral polio vaccine (Denmark, Israel and USA).[125]

Debate continues about the most appropriate vaccine to use, as each has important advantages and disadvantages. Inactivated polio vaccine has greatly reduced the spread of polio viruses in countries with small populations. And because there is no living virus in the vaccine, there is no possibility of it becoming virulent again. However, inactivated polio vaccine must be injected and it may not prevent intestinal infection. Also, the wild virus can circulate even in a population well-vaccinated with inactivated polio vaccine.[124] Live oral polio vaccine gives wider immunity as it behaves in a similar way to the natural infection. When the vaccine virus is passed in the stools, this leads to it spreading and displacing the wild virus in the community.[124] This may play a role in maintaining herd immunity by inadvertently immunising vulnerable people.

In the UK the use of inactivated polio vaccine in place of live oral polio has been considered, but it has been argued that the wild virus is a potential danger if inactivated polio vaccine alone is relied on for protection. This situation was illustrated recently in the Netherlands. Despite having high (97%) inactivated polio vaccine coverage in one-year olds, an epidemic of polio occurred in 1992–93 in the Netherlands among unimmunised people.[124] Some 71 patients were involved, with two deaths and 59 cases of paralysis. None of the patients had been immunised, and all but one belonged to a group of people who refuse vaccination for religious reasons. Other outbreaks have been documented among groups who refuse to be immunised with both inactivated polio vaccine and live oral polio vaccine programmes.[126]

A randomised, controlled trial was recently conducted in the UK to study the effects of giving infants a single dose of inactivated polio vaccine, followed by two doses of live oral polio vaccine. Results showed that, compared to the present schedule, a combined schedule would be likely to produce protection and is unlikely to greatly change the circulation of the polio virus in the community. It would also reduce the risk to those who had been given the vaccine.[124] As the global eradication of polio approaches, all countries will have to consider whether or not there is any longer a place for oral polio vaccine in immunisation schedules.

Adverse effects of live oral polio vaccine

The vaccine viruses may alter and rarely cause paralysis. Between 1985 and 1991, 54 suspected cases of polio were reported in England and Wales. Of these, 21 were confirmed to be caused by polio. Of these confirmed cases, 13 were associated with the vaccine – nine people had been given the vaccine themselves and four had been in contact with infants who had recently received their first dose of the oral polio vaccine. The other cases were imported from abroad.

From this information, the risk of vaccine-associated paralysis to those who are receiving the vaccine has been calculated at 1.46 in each million people for a first dose of vaccine, 0.49 of every million people for a second dose, zero for the third and fourth (booster) dose and 0.33 of every million people for the fifth (booster) dose.[127] The risk for contacts is more difficult to estimate as the number of contacts is not known. Assuming one contact per immunisation, the risk for unimmunised contacts would be 0.98 in every million people for the first dose and zero for the remaining doses, although in reality it is probably even lower than this. There would be no contact cases if all adults and children were immunised. It is important that anyone who has been in contact with recently vaccinated children knows of the need for strict personal hygiene, and particularly the importance of washing hands after changing nappies.

Despite the very small risk of vaccine-associated polio, oral polio vaccine is one of the safest and most effective vaccines used today.[127] However, because there are now so few cases of polio caused by the wild virus, it is inevitable that most cases will be associated with the vaccine.

In the early years of the production of polio vaccines, some were contaminated with a virus known as SV40. This virus, discovered in 1960, some years after polio vaccine had been introduced,[128] has been shown to cause tumours in rodents.[129] As soon as it was found in polio vaccine in 1961, measures were taken to ensure that no further contamination took place.[130] Oral polio virus became available in 1962. Stored samples of UK oral polio vaccine (dating back to 1966) have been tested and found to be free of the live SV40 virus (*personal communication* with Dr Philip Minor, National Institute for Biological Standards and Control).

Because it is known to cause cancer in some animals there was concern that it may also do so in humans. Although some researchers believe that they have found SV40 in some human tumour cells,[131-133] other researchers have not been able to confirm these findings.[134] Even if the virus is found in some tumours, this does not prove the virus causes them.[135] Two recent large studies have shown that people who received the polio vaccines contaminated with SV40 were no more likely to develop these particular cancers than those who received vaccine free of the virus.[136] There is no SV40 contamination of current polio vaccines.

Unvaccinated infants and swimming pools

Infants who have recently been given the oral polio vaccine, as well as those who are not immunised, can be taken swimming in public pools. Although the vaccine virus is shed in the water if babies defecate into the swimming pool, the dilution factor is so great in chlorinated water that it poses no risk.[137]

Effect of polio vaccination programmes

Polio was once a common disease with particularly large epidemics in the 1950s. (Figure 4 shows notifications of polio in England and Wales from 1920 to 1992.) In 1993, for the first time, there were fewer than 10,000 cases worldwide.[138] This was thanks to a combination of factors – routine immunisation, intensive surveillance and immunisation in response to outbreaks. It is claimed that the dramatic decline in polio cases following the introduction of vaccines in the 1950s was due to a refinement in how polio is diagnosed. As a result, conditions previously thought to be polio were categorised as other infections (for example, Coxsackie virus infections and aseptic meningitis).[139] If this were the case, a large increase in reports of these conditions could have been expected, but there is no evidence to suggest that this occurred.

Figure 4 Notifications of polio, England and Wales 1920–92

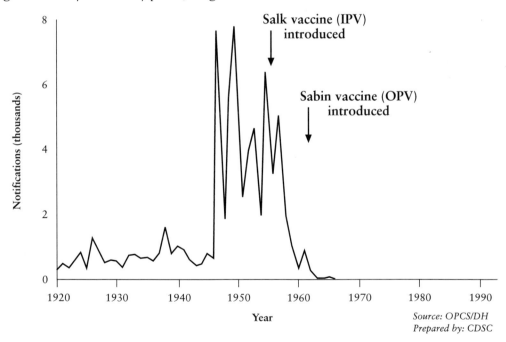

Source: OPCS/DH
Prepared by: CDSC

DIPHTHERIA

Diphtheria is an acute, highly infectious bacterial disease which mostly affects the upper respiratory tract, although the skin may also be affected.[140] A membrane forms over the respiratory tract, obstructing breathing and producing a powerful poison which causes tissue damage and attacks the heart and the nerves. Milder infections in those who are partially immune may lead to an uneventful recovery. Severe infections occur in the unimmunised and may lead to death.[4]

Incidence of diphtheria

Figures 5 and 6 show deaths and recorded cases of diphtheria from 1915. The number of deaths was declining before immunisation became available in 1942 (initially, it was directed towards children). In 1942 there were 41,404 recorded cases and 1827 deaths from the disease. By 1946 60% of children had been vaccinated and the number of deaths had fallen to 472.[141]

Figure 5 Diphtheria: registered deaths, England and Wales 1914–59

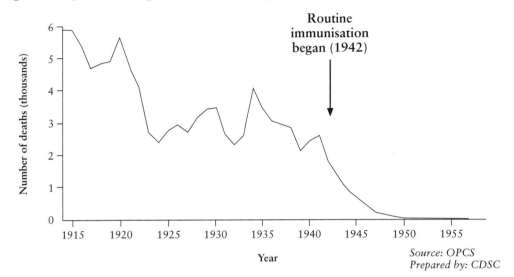

Source: OPCS
Prepared by: CDSC

Figure 6 Diphtheria: notifications, England and Wales 1914–59

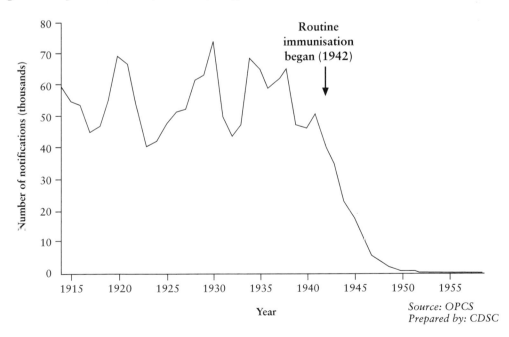

Source: OPCS
Prepared by: CDSC

In England and Wales diphtheria is now a rare disease, with only 13 cases and no deaths reported between 1986 and 1991, although in 1994 a 14-year-old boy who had recently returned from Pakistan died as a result of the disease.[142] An epidemic in the former USSR was reported in 1994, with some 47,802 cases and 1746 deaths.[143] Cases have been imported into countries that were previously free from this disease, demonstrating that it is important not to relax the control of diphtheria.[144]

Recent studies of immunity to diphtheria among adults in England have shown there to be decreasing immunity with increasing age. In addition, in the early years of diphtheria immunisation, uptake of the vaccine did not reach target levels (only 30% of babies were immunised by their first birthday in 1951–53). Overall results suggest that there are gaps in immunity among the adult population, with a third or more adults aged 35 years or over being susceptible to the infection. Diphtheria remains endemic in other countries, and the few cases that have been notified in this country in recent years have nearly all been imported, mostly from the Indian sub-continent, by unimmunised people. As Begg and Balraj point out, imported cases have not been responsible for any major outbreaks, but the potential does exist.[144] In an effort to improve adult immunity, immunisation of teenagers with low-dose diphtheria toxoid was started in October 1994.[145]

Diphtheria vaccine

Diphtheria vaccine contains the inactivated toxins from the organism. It is usually given with the tetanus and whooping cough vaccine. Common minor side effects of this immunisation include swelling and redness at the injection site. Malaise, fever and headache may also occur. More severe reactions to the vaccine are extremely uncommon.

TETANUS

When open wounds become contaminated with the tetanus organism, tetanus toxin is produced. This results in powerful muscle contractions. Death may result from obstruction in the respiratory tract.[4] Tetanus organisms are found everywhere and even a contaminated rose thorn prick can be enough to cause tetanus.[89] Being healthy and well nourished provides no protection against this disease.

Incidence of tetanus

The national tetanus immunisation programme began in 1961 and the disease has been virtually eliminated among children. Between 1985 and 1991 there were 104 cases of tetanus in England and Wales and 19 deaths. The highest risk group is women over 65 years, with a number of deaths following gardening injuries.[146] Studies have shown that the people most likely to have no immunity are over 50, and female. This may reflect the fact that more men have tetanus immunisation as a result of injuries, or routinely during military service.[146] (Tetanus immunisation has been provided by the armed forces since 1938.)[45]

Each individual needs to be given the tetanus vaccine as the disease is not spread from person to person and so there can be no herd immunity.

Tetanus vaccine

Tetanus vaccine contains the inactivated toxin from the organism. It is usually given with the diphtheria and whooping cough vaccine. Local reactions following vaccination such as pain, redness and swelling at the injection site may occur and persist for several days. General reactions are uncommon but include headaches, a fever and malaise. More severe reactions may occur and are more commonly associated with excessive use of the tetanus.[140] Booster doses are not recommended for immunised adults who have received five doses of the vaccine, except in the event of a probably contaminated wound, as booster doses have been shown to be unnecessary and can cause considerable local reactions. Cases of tetanus in individuals who were fully immunised many years previously have only occurred extremely rarely and have not proved fatal.[45]

TUBERCULOSIS (TB)

The TB organism usually enters through the respiratory tract during breathing. It causes a primary infection in the lung. Mild TB in children may be indistinguishable from a respiratory infection. In a few children there is direct spread within the lungs, the brain and spinal cord, bones, kidneys or other organs. Malnourished and unimmunised children are more likely to have the disease more severely.[4] TB of the central nervous system continues to be the most devastating form of the disease in childhood. Major after-effects in the nervous system follow in up to 70% of cases of meningitis, with reported death rates of 20%. Of the 5432 cases of TB reported in 1989, 10% occurred in children. TB meningitis accounted for less than 1% of the total cases, but 30% of these occurred in children.[147]

Prevalence of TB

Deaths from TB had been declining in England and Wales for at least 100 years.[148] However, in the late 1980s, reports of TB in England and Wales (plus other European countries and the USA) began to rise.[149] Incidences of TB are 20 to 30 times higher in people originating from the Indian subcontinent than in the white population here, and still higher in immigrants who have recently arrived. Recent studies have shown that TB continues to be strongly associated with poverty, and some of the recent increase in incidences has been put down to the expanding homeless population.

Bacille Calmette-Guérin (BCG) vaccine

Since it was introduced in the 1950s, routine BCG vaccination has played an important part in reducing TB in the UK. With the overall decline of TB, the number of vaccinations needed to prevent a single case of TB rose from 460 in 1969 to 2200 in 1984. It has been argued that the routine vaccination of school children is no longer cost-effective and could be stopped.[150] Indeed, despite guidelines by the Department of Health,[45] policies for BCG vaccination vary from district to district.

In ten randomised, controlled trials conducted throughout the world since the 1930s to determine the degree of protection of BCG vaccine, widely differing results (from 0 to 80%) have emerged. There is still no agreement on the reasons for this. Many factors are probably involved including the potency of the vaccine, the design of the study, age at vaccination, regional difference in the strain of TB organisms, and nutritional or genetic differences in the people involved in the trial.[147] However, the evidence for the vaccine's effectiveness in the UK is strong.[151] The Medical Research Council (MRC) trial of TB vaccine in England and Wales which began in 1950 showed that BCG vaccine given at age 14 was highly effective in preventing TB for at least 15 years.[147]

Only two of the trials assessed BCG given to newborn babies. Both trials were performed in North America and the effectiveness of the vaccine was estimated to be 75 to 80%. Case-control studies that have assessed BCG for the newborn have reported protection rates greater than 80%. This timing of BCG is particularly effective against the most severe form of the disease, TB meningitis, with an effectiveness of 85 to 100%.[147] Two studies of BCG given to newborn babies in England showed 64% and 75% protection respectively against generalised TB.[152,153]

Immunisation reaction

Normally, a reaction develops at the injection site within two to six weeks, beginning as a small pimple which increases in size for a few weeks. It widens into a circular area up to 7 mm in diameter with scaling, crusting and occasional bruising. This slowly subsides over several months and eventually heals leaving a small scar.[45]

Adverse reactions to BCG

Severe reactions at the injection site (such as large ulcers and abscesses) can occur but are most commonly caused by a faulty injection technique, where part or all of the dose is given too deeply.[45] Other complications following BCG immunisation are rare, although chronic ulceration and inflammation of the bone can occur in the newborn.[154] There have been reports of several cases of widely spread BCG in adults who were HIV positive at the time of immunisation. BCG should not be given to HIV positive people.[45]

HEPATITIS B

Infection with the hepatitis B virus can cause liver disease ranging from infection with no symptoms, acute self-limited hepatitis, up to fatal violent hepatitis. Infection, particularly when it occurs in early life, may result in an initially symptomless carrier state that can progress to chronic active hepatitis, cirrhosis of the liver and eventually cancer. Complex factors determine the outcome.[155] The hepatitis B virus is believed to be second only to tobacco among cancer-causing substances.[156] It is estimated that there are 400 to 500 million hepatitis B virus carriers in the world today.

Hepatitis B virus is present in various body fluids including blood, saliva, semen, vaginal fluid and breast milk. These fluids may be highly infectious. The disease can be spread by sexual intercourse and from mother to child, both at birth and while breastfeeding.[157] Babies born to mothers carrying hepatitis B antigen have an 80 to 90% risk of becoming infected immediately before and after birth and a 40% risk of death from hepatitis B-associated cirrhosis or cancer in later life. Babies born to mothers who have developed their own antibodies to hepatitis B are at a much lower risk.[158]

Incidence of hepatitis B in the UK

The frequency of hepatitis B infection in this country is not certain. Antenatal clinics in certain inner city areas report that up to 1 in 100 women carry hepatitis B.[45] The number of cases of hepatitis in the UK is low and, along with other countries in Northern and Western Europe, the UK is ranked as being a low-prevalence country.[159]

Hepatitis B vaccine

The vaccine currently used is genetically engineered. The older vaccine (which was derived from blood plasma) is no longer marketed in the UK. Response rates to the vaccine are close to 100% in healthy young adults, children and newborn babies,[156] although immunity decreases with age, particularly in those over the age of 40.[160] It is not known yet whether a course of hepatitis B vaccine given to children will provide lifelong immunity. However, long-term studies should show whether booster doses of the vaccine are needed.[161]

Adverse effects of hepatitis B vaccine

In the USA, vaccine-related adverse events are reported to the Vaccine Adverse Event Reporting System by vaccine manufacturers, health care providers and the public. Events known to be linked in cause to a vaccine, as well as all events related in time to when a vaccine is given, are reported. In a study of the safety of hepatitis B vaccine among newborn babies and young children over a four-year period (1991–94), fever was the most common serious symptom reported.[162] There were also reports of agitation, discolouration of the skin, convulsions and temporarily stopping breathing.

The limitations of a passive reporting system include the fact that it does not show whether a vaccine caused the adverse effect. Information on the number of people vaccinated is also lacking. This makes it impossible to calculate rates for the vaccine-related events, and so to be able to compare them with the rate of these events in a non-immunised population. However, during this time, at least 12 million doses of vaccine were given to the age groups of interest.

Hepatitis B vaccination policy

Due to the high risks attached to this infection, it is becoming common in the UK for pregnant women to be screened for the hepatitis B virus. Babies of infected mothers are vaccinated at birth, and also at 1 month and 6 months of age. In the USA, universal immunisation of all infants has been recommended,[163] mainly with the aim of preventing the infection in adolescents and adults. An alternative option would be universal vaccination in early adolescence. This would be effective in preventing adolescent hepatitis B virus infection, but would not prevent transmission in early childhood, when the risk of developing complications is highest.[164] In Italy, both options have been adopted. In this country the debate about the most appropriate vaccination policy continues. Although the prevalence is low, the severity of the disease makes it one of the most serious infectious diseases in Europe.[159]

NEW VACCINES

Vaccine technology is a rapidly developing field. It is likely that new vaccines will be introduced before the end of the decade. Possible vaccines include varicella (chicken-pox) vaccine, respiratory syncitial virus vaccine, rotavirus vaccine and vaccines that protect against other forms of bacterial meningitis. In addition, a great deal of work is being devoted to improving existing vaccines, such as the whooping cough vaccine. Genetic engineering is helping in the production of vaccines.[165]

Most vaccines in current use (except the oral polio vaccine) are injected. New approaches to immunisation are being introduced, such as ways of giving more vaccines without injections. This is being investigated in the case of several viruses and it is hoped that a longer-lasting immunity similar to that following natural infection may be achieved.[166]

It is also desirable for vaccines to be developed by methods that will allow greater control of their biological properties in order to eliminate their side effects as far as possible.[167] Other desirable properties include vaccines with greater heat stability (particularly for use in non-industrialised countries) and vaccines in which several antigens can be given by a single injection.

CONCLUSIONS

There is little doubt that, in combination with other public health measures, immunisation programmes have been successful in reducing the incidence of disease and related deaths worldwide. However, to individual parents deciding whether to have their child immunised, this fact may be of little relevance. One of the consequences of a successful immunisation programme is that it may result in parents believing that their children are not at risk of disease and dwelling on the potential risks of the vaccine instead. This belief is fed by well-publicised stories of individual children who developed problems following immunisation and by non-mainstream publications that claim to provide sound evidence against immunisation.

It is clear that when immunisation levels go down, disease levels rise which places individual children as well as populations at risk. No vaccine can be guaranteed 100% safe, but the chances of a child being seriously and permanently damaged as a result of vaccination are remote. On the other hand, the risk of complications and death associated with infectious disease is significant. It is this fact that should be considered very carefully when making a decision about immunisation. It is necessary to keep vaccination uptake high to make sure that individual children as well as the whole community continue to be protected from infectious disease.

Explanation of terms used

Acellular not containing cells. Acellular vaccine does not contain the killed bacteria cells.

Adjuvant a substance which, when mixed with an antigen, increases the immune response.

Anaphylaxis a serious form of allergic reaction where the following symptoms may develop: pallor, limpness and difficulty in breathing, upper airway obstruction, severe slowing of the pulse, and rapid development of a skin reaction marked by the development of itchy or burning wheals. This can result in heart failure and sometimes death.

Antibody a protein produced as a result of the presence of an antigen (either by natural infection or by immunisation) and which fights infection.

Antigen a substance which, under appropriate conditions, triggers an immune response. Vaccines are specially-prepared antigens.

Apnoea temporary absence or stoppage of breathing.

Arthralgia pain in a joint.

Asymptomatic infection infection with no symptoms.

Auto immune disease auto immunity is the process whereby an individual develops antibodies which attack his or her own tissues. An individual does not normally develop antibodies which attack his or her own tissues, but only to foreign cells such as micro-organisms.

Clinical infection infection with symptoms.

Crohn's disease an inflammatory bowel disease.

Encephalitis inflammation of the brain.

Encephalopathy a general term to cover any degenerative or non-inflammatory disease of the brain.

Guillain-Barré syndrome (GBS) a condition which usually follows a viral or bacterial infection. Symptoms are general weakness or paralysis, frequently affecting respiratory as well as peripheral muscles.

Immunisation	the introduction of a substance, usually a vaccine, which causes the production of antibodies in the body.
Immunity	a principle by which a person is protected from certain diseases or the action of certain poisons.
Immunodeficiency	a reduction in a person's natural immunity affecting their ability to fight infections.
Infectious	any disease, or condition attributable to infection or to an infectious agent. When applied to an individual it means they are in a state to transmit an infection either by direct contact or indirectly (for example by an insect such as in malaria)
Meninges	the membranes that enclose the brain and spinal cord.
Respiratory syncitial	the main cause of bronchiolitis (inflammation of the small
virus	tubes in the lungs) and pneumonia in babies
Rotavirus	the main cause of gastroenteritus (diarrhoea and vomiting) in young children throughout the world
Subacute sclerosing panencephalitis (SSPE)	a rare, late complication of natural measles infection, caused by the measles virus being reactivated after lying dormant. The period between measles and the onset of SSPE is usually about seven years. Initial signs include loss of intellectual abilities, followed by lack of coordination. The condition is usually fatal.
Vaccination	the process of active immunisation with any vaccine in order to produce immunity. In practice the terms vaccination and immunisation are interchangeable.
Whole-cell vaccine	a vaccine containing whole, killed organisms.

References

1 INTRODUCTION: THE IMMUNISATION DECISION

1. Health Education Authority. *Guide to childhood immunisations*. 1998. HEA, London.

2. Department of Health. *Immunisation against infectious disease*. 1996. HMSO, London.

3. Neustaedter, R. 'The immunization decision', *The Family Health Series*. 1990. North Atlantic Books, Berkeley.

4. What Doctors Don't Tell You. *The WDDTY vaccination handbook*. What Doctors Don't Tell You. 1991. The Wallace Press, London.

5. Coulter, H.L. 'Vaccination and sociopathy', *International Journal of Alternative and Complementary Medicine*, 1992; October: 12–15.

6. Gunn, T. *Mass immunisation: a point in question*. 1992. Cutting Edge Publications, Ulverston, Cumbria.

7. Scheibner, V. *Vaccination – 100 years of orthodox research shows that vaccines represent a medical assault on the immune system*. 1993. Australian Print Group, Victoria.

8. Wade, D. 'Vaccines; lifesaving jab or shot in the dark?', *Independent on Sunday*, 1991; 8 September.

9. Thomas, T. 'Why child vaccine may be a shot in the dark', *Independent*, 1993; 9 February.

10. Roberts, Y. 'A shot in the dark', *Sunday Times*, 1995; December.

2 IMMUNITY

1. Mortimer, E.A. 'Pertussis vaccines', in Plotkin, S.A., Mortimer, E.A. (eds) *Vaccines*. 1994. W.B. Saunders, Philadelphia.

2. Feigin, R.D., Cherry, J.D. 'Pertussis', in *Textbook of pediatric infectious diseases*. 1981. W.B. Saunders, Philadelphia.

3. Howie, P.W., Forsyth, J.S., Ogston, S.A., Clark, A., Florey, C.D. 'Protective effect of breast feeding against infection', *British Medical Journal*, 1990; 300: 11–16.

4. Aniansson, G., Alm, B., Andersson, B., Hakansson, A., Larsson, P., Nylen, O. 'A prospective cohort study on breast-feeding and otitis media in Swedish infants', *Pediatric Infectious Disease Journal*, 1994; 13: 183–8.

5. Beaudry, M., Dufour, R., Marcoux, S. 'Relation between infant feeding and infections during the first six months of life', *The Journal of Pediatrics*, 1995; 126(2): 191–7.

6. Shapiro, E.D., Ward, J.I. 'The epidemiology and prevention of disease caused by *Haemophilus influenzae* type b', *Epidemiologic Reviews*, 1991; 13: 113–42.

7. Cunningham, A.S. 'Breast-feeding and morbidity in industrialized countries: an update', in Jelliffe, D.B & E.F.P. (eds) *Advances in international maternal and child health*. Volume 1. 1981. Oxford University Press, Oxford.

8. Riordan, J., Auerbach, K.G. 'The biologic specificity of breastmilk', in *Breastfeeding and human lactation*. 1993. Jones & Bartlett, Boston.

9. Newman, J. 'How breastmilk protects newborns', *Scientific American*, 1995; December: 58–61.

10. Bellanti, J.A. 'Basic immunologic principles underlying vaccination procedures', *Pediatric Clinics of North America*, 1990; 37(3): 513–30.

11. Mortimer, E.A. 'Communicable diseases', in Pless, I.B. (ed.) *The epidemiology of childhood disorders*. 1994. Oxford University Press, Oxford.

12. Sutter, R.W., Markowitz, L.E., Bennetch, J.M., Morris, W., Zell, E.R., Preblud, S.R. 'Measles among the Amish: a comparative study of measles severity in primary and secondary cases in households', *The Journal of Infectious Diseases*, 1991; 163: 12–16.

13. Center for Disease Control. 'Isolation of wild poliovirus type 3 among members of a religious community objecting to vaccination – Alberta, Canada, 1993', *Mortality and Morbidity Weekly Report*, 1993; 42: 337–9.

14. Miller, C.L. 'Deaths from measles in England and Wales, 1970–83', *British Medical Journal*, 1985; 290: 443–4.

15. Watson, R.R. 'Nutrition and immunity', *Modern Medicine*, 1982; November: 25–7.

16. McTaggart, L. *What doctors don't tell you*. 1996. Thorsons, London.

17. Frieden, T.R., Sowell, A.L., Henning, K.J., Huff, D.L., Gunn, R.A. 'Vitamin A levels and severity of measles', *American Journal of Diseases in Children*, 1992; 146: 182–6.

18. Gunn, T. 'Measles and immunity', *The Informed Parent*, 1994; 9.

19. English, J.M. 'The rights and wrongs of measles vaccination', *British Homeopathic Journal*, 1995; 84: 156-63.

20. Curtis, S. *A handbook of homeopathic alternatives to immunisation*. 1994. Winter Press, London.

21. Gellin, B.G., Katz, S.L. 'Measles: state of the art and future directions', *The Journal of Infectious Diseases*, 1994; 170(suppl. 1): S3–14.

22. Shaheen, S.O., Aaby, P., Hall, A.J., Barker, D.J.P., Heyes, C.B., Shiell, A.W., Goudiaby, A. 'Cell mediated immunity after measles in Guinea-Bissau: historical cohort study', *British Medical Journal*, 1996; 313: 969–74.

23. Cutts, F.T., Markowitz, L.E. 'Successes and failures in measles control', *The Journal of Infectious Diseases*, 1994; 170(suppl.): S32–41.

24. Miller, C.L., Fletcher, W.B. 'Severity of notified whooping cough', *British Medical Journal*, 1976; 1: 117–19.

25. James, J.M., Burks, A.W., Roberson, P.K., Sampson, H.A. 'Safe administration of the measles vaccine to children allergic to eggs', *The New England Journal of Medicine*, 1995; 332: 1262–6.

26. Aickin, R., Hill, D., Kemp, A. 'Measles immunisation in children with allergy to egg', *British Medical Journal*, 1994; 309: 223–5.

27. King, P.F., Perl, D.P., Brieree, L.M. *et al.* 'Selective accumulation of aluminium and iron in the neurofibrillary tangles of Alzheimer's disease', *Annals of Neurology*, 1992; 31: 286–92.

28. Martyn, C.N., Osmond, C., Edwardson, J.A. *et al.* 'Geographical relationship between Alzheimer's disease and the aluminium in drinking water', *The Lancet*, 1989; i: 59–62.

29. Southgate, D.A.T. 'Any questions?', *British Medical Journal*, 1989; 298: 1172.

3 INFORMATION ABOUT IMMUNISATION

1. Shapiro, E.D., Ward, J.I. 'The epidemiology and prevention of disease caused by *Haemophilus influenzae* type b', *Epidemiologic Reviews*, 1991; 13: 113–42.

2. Jones, D.M., Kaczmarski, E.B. 'Meningococcal infections in England and Wales: 1994', *Communicable Disease Report*, 1995; R5 (9): R125–R129.

3. Begg, N.T., Cutts, F.T. 'The role of epidemiology in the development of a vaccination programme', in *Vaccination and World Health*. 1994. John Wiley & Sons, Chichester.

4. Paradiso, P.R., Hogerman, D.A., Madore, D.V., Keyserling, H., King, J., Reisinger, K.S. 'Safety and immunogenicity of a combined diphtheria, tetanus, pertussis and *Haemophilus influenzae* type b vaccine in young infants', *Pediatrics*, 1993; 92(6): 827–32.

5. Dudgeon, J.A., Cutting, W.A.M. (eds) *Immunization: principles and practice*. 1991. Chapman & Hall Medical, London.

6. Ramsey, M.E.B., Gay, N., Miller, E., Rush, M., White, J., Morgan-Capner, P., Brown, D. 'The epidemiology of measles in England and Wales: rationale for the 1994 national vaccination campaign', *Communicable Disease Report*, 1994; R12(4): R141–146.

7. Center for Disease Control and Prevention. 'Update: vaccine side effects, adverse reactions, contraindications, and precautions – recommendations of the Advisory Committee on Immunization Practices (ACIP)', *Morbidity and Mortality Weekly Report*, 1996; 45 (RR–12).

8. Fulginiti, V.A. 'Sudden infant death syndrome, diphtheria-tetanus-toxoid-pertussis vaccination and visits to the doctor: chance association or cause and effect?', *Pediatric Infectious Diseases*, 1983; 2(1): 5–6.

9. Department of Health. *Immunisation against infectious disease*. 1996. HMSO, London.

10. Maguire, H.C., Begg, N.T., Handford, S.G. 'Meningoencephalitis associated with MMR vaccine', *Communicable Disease Report*, 1991; 1: R60–R61.

11. Farrington, P., Pugh, S., Colville, A., Flower, A., Nash, J., Morgan-Capner, P. *et al.* 'A new method for active surveillance of adverse events from diphtheria/tetanus/pertussis and measles/mumps/rubella vaccines', *The Lancet*, 1995; 345: 567–9.

4 THE EFFECT IMMUNISATION PROGRAMMES HAVE ON THE INCIDENCE OF INFECTIOUS DISEASES

1. Scheibner, V. *Vaccination – 100 years of orthodox research shows that vaccines represent a medical assault on the immune system*. 1993. Australian Print Group, Victoria.

2. Peter, G. (ed.) *Report of the Committee on Infectious Diseases*, 1994. American Academy of Pediatrics, Illinois.

3. Department of Health. PL CMO (94)2. *Meningococcal infection: meningitis and septicaemia*. 1994. HMSO, London.

4. Department of Health. *Immunisation against infectious disease*. 1996. HMSO, London.

5. White, J.M., Fairley, C.K., Owen, D., Matthews, R.C., Miller, E. 'The effect of an accelerated immunisation schedule on pertussis in England and Wales', *Communicable Disease Report*, 1996; 6: R86–R91.

6. Pollard, R. 'Relation between vaccination and notification rates for whooping cough in England and Wales', *The Lancet*, 1980; ii: 1180–2.

7. Bloch, A.B., Orenstein, W.A., Stetler, H.C., Wassilak, S.G., Amler, R.W., Bart, K.J. *et al.* 'Health impact of measles vaccination in the United States', *Pediatrics*, 1985; 76: 524–32.

8. Brown, D.W.G., Ramsey, M.E.B., Richards, A.F., Miller, E. 'Salivary diagnosis of measles: a study of notified cases in the United Kingdom, 1991–3', *British Medical Journal*, 1994; 308: 1015–17.

9. Lennon, J.L., Black, F.L. 'Maternally derived measles immunity in an era of vaccine-protected mothers', *Journal of Pediatrics*, 1986; 671–6.

10. Brugha, R., Ramsey, M., Forsey, T., Brown, D. 'A study of maternally derived measles antibody in infants born to naturally infected and vaccinated women', *Epidemiology and Infection*, 1996: 117: 519–24.

11. Miller, E., Marshall, R., Vurdien, J. 'Epidemiology, outcome and control of varicella-zoster infection', *Reviews in Medical Microbiology*, 1993; 4: 222–30.

12. What Doctors Don't Tell You. *The WDDTY vaccination handbook*. *What Doctors Don't Tell You*. 1991. The Wallace Press, London.

13. Cutts, F.T., Markowitz, L.E. 'Successes and failures in measles control', *The Journal of Infectious Diseases*, 1994; 170(suppl.): S32–41.

5 GENERAL ISSUES

1. Curtis, S. *A handbook of homeopathic alternatives to immunisation*. 1994. Winter Press, London.

2. Rogers, A., Pilgrim, D. 'Non-compliance with childhood immunisation: personal accounts of parents and primary health care professionals', Unpublished.

3. Forrest, J. *Who calls the shots? An analysis of lay beliefs about childhood vaccination*. Occasional Papers in Sociology and Social Policy No. 3, 1995. South Bank University, London.

4. Alderson, P., Mayall, B., Barker, S., Henderson, J., Pratten, B. 'Childhood immunisation: meeting targets yet respecting consent', *The European Journal of Public Health*, 1997; 7: 95–100.

5. Miller, E., Goldacre, M., Pugh, S., Colville, A., Farrington, P., Flower, A. *et al.* 'Risk of aseptic meningitis after measles, mumps and rubella vaccine in UK children', *The Lancet*, 1993; 341: 979–82.

6. Ramsey, M.E.B., Rao, M., Begg, N.T. 'Symptoms after accelerated immunisation', *British Medical Journal*, 1992; 304: 1534–6.

7. Farrington, P., Pugh, S., Colville, A., Flower, A., Nash, J., Morgan-Capner, P. *et al.* 'A new method for active surveillance of adverse events from diphtheria/tetanus/pertussis and measles/mumps/rubella vaccines', *The Lancet*, 1995; 345: 567–9.

8. Ramsey, M.E.B., Rao, M., Begg, N.T., Redhead, K., Attwell, A-M. 'Antibody response to accelerated immunisation with diphtheria, tetanus, pertussis vaccine', *The Lancet*, 1993; 342: 203–5.

9. Ramsey, M.E.B., Corbel, M.J., Redhead, K., Ashworth, L.A.E., Begg, N.T. 'Persistence of antibody after accelerated immunisation with diphtheria/tetanus/pertussis vaccine', *British Medical Journal*, 1991; 302: 1489–91.

10. Pullan, C. 'Routine immunisation of preterm infants', *Archives of Disease in Childhood*, 1989; 64: 1438–41.

11. Bellanti, J.A. 'Basic immunologic principles underlying vaccination procedures', *Pediatric Clinics of North America*, 1990; 37(3): 513–30.

12. Smolen, P., Bland, R., Heiligenstein, E. *et al.* 'Antibody response to oral polio vaccine in premature infants', *The Journal of Pediatrics*, 1983; 103: 917–19.

13. Bernbaum, J., Daft, A., Anolik, R. *et al.* 'Response of preterm infants to diphtheria–tetanus–pertussis immunizations', *The Journal of Pediatrics*, 1985: 107: 184–8.

14. Koblin, B.A., Townsend, T.R., Munoz, A., Onorato, I., Wilson, M., Polk, B.F. 'Response of preterm infants to diphtheria-tetanus-pertussis vaccine', *Pediatric Infectious Disease Journal*, 1988; 7: 704–11.

15. Conway, S., James, J., Balfour, A., Smithells, R. 'Immunisation of the pre-term baby', *Journal of Infection*, 1993; 27: 143–50.

6 EXPERIENCES OF IMMUNISATION AND INFECTIOUS DISEASES IN OTHER COUNTRIES

1. Hinman, A.R., Orenstein, W.A. 'Immunization practice in developed countries', in Moxon, R.E. (ed.) *Modern vaccines: a Lancet review*. 1990. Edward Arnold, London.

2. Roberts, L. 'Needle points', *Guardian*, 1995; 21 March.

3. Romanus, V., Jonsell, R., Bergquist, S.-O. 'Pertussis in Sweden after the cessation of general immunisation in 1979', *Pediatric Infectious Disease Journal*, 1987; 6: 364–71.

4. Rattigan, P. *Vaccine legacy*. 1994. Chesterfield.

5. Oda, M., Higurashi, M. 'Development of acellular pertussis vaccine in Japan', *Acta Paediatrica Japonica*, 1988; 30: 136–42.

6. Kimura, M., Kuno-Sakai, H. 'Pertussis vaccines in Japan', *Acta Paediatrica Japonica*, 1988; 30: 143–53.

7. Mortimer, E.A. 'Communicable diseases', in Pless, I.B. (ed.) *The epidemiology of childhood disorders*. 1994. Oxford University Press, Oxford.

8. Kimura, M., Kuno-Sakai, H. 'Developments in pertussis immunisation in Japan', *The Lancet*, 1990; 336: 30–1.

9. Ueda, K., Miyazaki, C., Hidaka, Y., Okada, K., Kusuhara, K., Kadoya, R. 'Aseptic meningitis caused by measles-mumps-rubella vaccine in Japan', *The Lancet*, 1995; 346: 701-702.

10. Binkin, N.J., Samaso, S., Tozzi, A.E., Scuderi, G., Greco, D. 'Epidemiology of pertussis in a developed country with low vaccination coverage: the Italian experience', *Pediatric Infectious Disease Journal*, 1992; 11: 653–61.

11. Miller, E., Farrington, C.P. 'The current epidemiology of pertussis in the developed world: UK and West Germany', *Tokai Journal of Experimental and Clinical Medicine*, 1988; 13(suppl.): 97–101.

12. What Doctors Don't Tell You. *The WDDTY vaccination handbook*. What Doctors Don't Tell You, 1991. The Wallace Press, London.

13. Center for Disease Control. 'Standards for pediatric immunization practices', *Morbidity and Mortality Weekly Report*, 1993; 42 (RR-5): 1–13.

14. Atkinson, W.L., Orenstein, W.A. 'The resurgence of measles in the United States, 1989–1990', *Annual Reviews of Medicine*, 1992; 43: 451–63.

15. Anders, J.F., Jacobson, R.M., Poland, G.A., Jacobsen, S.J., Wollan, P.C. 'Secondary failure rates of measles vaccine: a metaanalysis of published studies', *Pediatric Infectious Disease Journal*, 1996; 15: 62–6.

16. Center for Disease Control. 'Measles – United States, 1995', *Morbidity and Mortality Weekly Report*, 1996; 45(15): 305–7.

17. Center for Disease Control. 'Measles – United States, first 26 weeks, 1994', *Morbidity and Mortality Weekly Report*, 1994; 43(37): 673–6.

18. Peltola, H., Heinonen, O.P., Valle, M., Paunio, M., Virtanen, M., Karanko, V. 'The elimination of indigenous measles, mumps and rubella from Finland by a 12-year, two-dose vaccination program', *The New England Journal of Medicine*, 1994; 331(21): 1397–1402.

7 ALTERNATIVES TO IMMUNISATION

1. Neustaedter, R. 'The immunization decision', *The Family Health Series*. 1990. North Atlantic Books, Berkeley.

2. Neustaedter, R. 'Measles and homeopathic immunisations', *The Homeopath*, 1990; 10(2): 31–2, 42.

3. English, J. 'The issue of immunization', *British Homeopathic Journal*, 1992; 81: 161–3.

4. Fisher, P. 'Enough nonsense on immunization', *British Homeopathic Journal*, 1990; 79: 198–200.

5. English, J.M. 'Pertussin 30 – preventive for whooping cough?', *British Homeopathic Journal*, 1987; 76: 61–5.

6. Bellanti, J.A. 'Basic immunologic principles underlying vaccination procedures', *Pediatric Clinics of North America*, 1990; 37(3): 513–30.

7. Smolen, P., Bland, R., Heiligenstein, E. *et al*. 'Antibody response to oral polio vaccine in premature infants', *The Journal of Pediatrics*, 1983; 103: 917–19.

8. Bernbaum, J.,Daft, A., Anolik, R. *et al*. 'Response of preterm infants to diphtheria–tetanus–pertussis immunizations', *The Journal of Pediatrics*, 1985; 107: 184–8.

9. Ramsey, M.E.B., Rao, M., Begg, N.T., Redhead, K., Attwell, A.-M. 'Antibody response to accelerated immunisation with diphtheria, tetanus, pertussis vaccine', *The Lancet*, 1993; 342: 203–5.

8 SPECIFIC CONDITIONS THAT HAVE BEEN CLAIMED TO BE LINKED TO IMMUNISATION

1. Scheibner, V. *Vaccination – 100 years of orthodox research shows that vaccines represent a medical assault on the immune system*. 1993. Australian Print Group, Victoria.

2. Gilbert, R. 'The changing epidemiology of SIDS', *Archives of Disease in Childhood*', 1994; 70: 445–9.

3. Nicoll, A., Gardner, A. 'Whooping cough and unrecognised postperinatal mortality', *Archives of Disease in Childhood*, 1988; 63: 41–7.

4. Howson, C.P., Howe, C. J. and Fineberg, H.V (eds.). *Adverse effects of pertussis and rubella vaccines*. 1991. National Academy Press, Washington.

5. Bouvier-Colle, M.H., Flahaut, A., Messiah, A., Jougla, E., Hatton, F. 'Sudden infant death and immunization: an extensive epidemiological approach to the problem in France', *International Journal of Epidemiology*, 1986; 18: 121–6.

6. Pollock, T.M., Mortimer, J.Y., Miller, E., Smith, G. 'Symptoms after primary immunisation with DTP and DT vaccine', *The Lancet*, 1984; 2: 146–9.

7. Taylor, E.M., Emery, J.L. 'Immunisation and cot deaths' (letter), *The Lancet*, 1982; 2: 721.

8. Hoffman, H.J., Hunter, J.C., Damus, K., Pakter, J., Peterson, D.R., van Belle, G. *et al*. 'Diphtheria-tetanus-pertussis immunization and sudden infant death: results of child health and human development cooperative epidemiological study of sudden infant death syndrome risk factors', *Pediatrics*, 1987; 79(4): 598–611.

9. Walker, A.M., Jick, H., Perara, D.R., Thompson, R.S., Knauss, T.A. 'Diphtheria-tetanus-pertussis immunization and sudden death syndrome', *American Journal of Public Health*, 1987; 77: 945–51.

10. Griffin, M.R., Ray, W.A., Livengood, J.R., Scaffner, W. 'Risk of sudden infant death syndrome after immunization with the diphtheria-tetanus-pertussis vaccine', *The New England Journal of Medicine*, 1988; 2: 618–23.

11. Solberg, L.K. 'DTP vaccination, visits to child health centers and sudden infant death syndrome (SIDS)', 1985. Report to the Oslo Health Council.

12. Mitchell, E.A., Stewart, A.W., Clements, M., Ford, R.P.K. 'Immunisation and the sudden infant death syndrome', *Archives of Disease in Childhood*, 1995; 73: 498–501.

13. Noble, G.R., Bernier, R.H., Esber, E.C., Hardegree, C., Hinman, A.R., Klein, D. 'Acellular and whole-cell pertussis vaccines in Japan', *Journal of the American Medical Association*, 1987; 257(10): 1351–6.

14. Office of Population Censuses and Surveys, DH3 94/1. 'Sudden infant deaths, 1989–93', *OPCS Monitor*, 1994; 15 December.

15. Center for Disease Control. 'Diphtheria, tetanus and pertussis: Guidelines for vaccine prophylaxis and other preventive measures', *Morbidity and Mortality Weekly Report*, 1981; 30: 392–6, 401–7.

16. Corne, J. 'Any questions?', *British Medical Journal*, 1994; 309: 1001.

17. Odent, M.R., Culpin, E.E., Kimmel, T. 'Pertussis vaccination and asthma: is there a link?' (letter), *Journal of the American Medical Association*, 1994; 272(8): 592–3.

18. The Informed Parent. 'Breastfed babies study', *The Informed Parent*, 1993; October: 5:2.

19. Lewis, C. 'GP data cast doubt over pertussis link in asthma', *Pulse*, 1994; 8 October.

20. Nilsson, L., Kjellman, N.-I.M., Storsaeter, J., Gustafsson, L., Olin, P. 'Lack of association between pertussis vaccination and symptoms of asthma and allergy', *Journal of the American Medical Association*, 1996; 275(10): 760.

21. Butler, N.R., Golding, J. (eds) *From birth to five*. 1986. Pergamon Press, Oxford.

22. Butler, N.R., Golding, J., Haslum, M., Stewart-Brown, S. 'Recent findings from the 1970 child health and education study: preliminary communication', *Journal of the Royal Society of Medicine*, 1982; 75: 781–4.

23. Pollock, J.I. *Completing the primary vaccination course*. 1991. Unpublished report for the Health Promotion Trust. 1991.

24. Coulter, H.L. 'Vaccination and sociopathy', *International Journal of Alternative and Complementary Medicine*, 1992; October: 12–15.

25. Fisher, P. 'Enough nonsense on immunization', *British Homeopathic Journal*, 1990; 79: 198–200.

26. Stiller, C.A. 'Malignancies', in Pless, I.B. *The epidemiology of childhood disorders*. 1994. Oxford University Press, Oxford.

27. Kneale, G.W., Stewart, A.M., Kinnier-Wilson, L.M. 'Immunizations against infectious diseases and childhood cancers', *Cancer Immunology and Immunotherapy*, 1986; 21: 129–32.

28. Hartley, A.L., Birch, J.M., McKinney, P.A., Blair, V., Teare, M.D., Carrette, J., *et al.* 'The inter-regional epidemiological study of childhood cancer (IRESCC); past medical history in children with cancer', *Journal of Epidemiology and Community Health*, 1988; 42: 235–42.

29. Christie, A.B. 'Measles', in *Infectious diseases: epidemiology and clinical practice*. 1980. Churchill Livingstone, Edinburgh.

30. Svenningsson, A. *et al.* 'Incidence of MS during two 15 year periods in the Gothenburg region of Sweden', *Acta Neurologica Scandinavica*, 1990; 161–8.

31. Gellin, B.G., Katz, S.L. 'Measles: state of the art and future directions', *The Journal of Infectious Diseases*, 1994; 170(suppl. 1): S3–14.

32. Cherry, J.D., Feigin, R.D., Lobes, L.A., Shackelford, P.G. 'Atypical measles in children previously immunized with attenuated measles virus vaccines', *Pediatrics*, 1972; 50(5): 712–17.

33. Miller, E., Marshall, R., Vurdien, J. 'Epidemiology, outcome and control of varicella-zoster infection', *Reviews in Medical Microbiology*, 1993; 4: 222–30.

34. Farrington, C. P. 'Subacute sclerosing panencephalitis in England and Wales: transient effects and risk estimates,' *Statistics in Medicine*, 1991; 10: 1733–44.

35. Miller, C., Farrington, C.P., Harbert, K. 'The epidemiology of subacute sclerosing panencephalitis in England and Wales 1970–1989', *International Journal of Epidemiology*, 1992; 21(5): 998–1006.

36. Plotkin, S.A., Starr, S., Connor, K., Morton, D. 'Zoster in normal children after varicella vaccine,' *Journal of Infectious Diseases*, 1989; 159: 1000.

37. Feldman, S., Hughes, W. T., Kim, H.Y. 'Herpes zoster in children with cancer,' *American Journal of Diseases of Children*, 1973; 126: 178–184.

38. Brunell, P. A., Taylor-Wiedeman, J., Geiser, C.F., Fierson, L., Lydick, E. 'Risk of herpes zoster in children with leukaemia: varicella vaccine compared with history of chicken pox,' *Pediatrics*, 1986; 77: 53–6.

39. Hardy, I., Gershon, A.A., Steinberg, S.P., LaRussa, P. 'The incidence of zoster after immunization with live attenuated varicella vaccine,' *New England Journal of Medicine*, 1991; 325 (22): 1545–1550.

9 THE DISEASES AND VACCINES

1. Dudgeon, J.A. 'Measles vaccines', *British Medical Journal*, 1969; 25(2): 153–8.

2. Miller, C.L. 'Deaths from measles in England and Wales, 1970–83', *British Medical Journal*, 1985; 290: 443–4.

3. Miller, C.L. 'Convulsions after measles vaccination' (letter), *The Lancet*, 1983; 2: 215.

4. Davies, E.G., Elliman, D.A.C., Hart, C.A., Nicoll, A., Rudd, P.T. *Manual of childhood infections.* 1996. W.B. Saunders, London.

5. Bloch, A.B., Orenstein, W.A., Stetler, H.C., Wassilak, S.G., Amler, R.W., Bart, K.J. *et al.* 'Health impact of measles vaccination in the United States', *Pediatrics*, 1985; 76: 524–32.

6. Markowitz, L.E., Orenstein, W.A. 'Measles vaccines', *Pediatric Clinics of North America*, 1990; 37(3): 603–25.

7. Miller, C., Farrington, C.P., Harbert, K. 'The epidemiology of subacute sclerosing panencephalitis in England and Wales 1970–1989', *International Journal of Epidemiology*, 1992; 21(5): 998–1006.

8. Miller, C. 'Live measles vaccine: a 21 year follow up', *British Medical Journal*, 1987; 295: 22–4.

9. Ramsey, M.E.B., Moffatt, D., O'Connor, M. 'Measles vaccine: a 27 year follow-up', *Epidemiology and Infection*, 1994; 112: 409–12.

10. Markowitz, L.E., Preblud, S.R., Fine, P.E.M., Orenstein, W.A. 'Duration of live measles vaccine-induced immunity', *Pediatric Infectious Disease Journal*, 1990; 9(2): 101–10.

11. Gellin, B.G., Katz, S.L. 'Measles: state of the art and future directions', *The Journal of Infectious Diseases*, 1994; 170(suppl. 1): S3–14.

12. Miller, C.L. 'Surveillance after measles vaccination in children', *The Practitioner*, 1982; 226: 535–7.

13. Farrington, P., Pugh, S., Colville, A., Flower, A., Nash, J., Morgan-Capner, P. *et al.* 'A new method for active surveillance of adverse events from diphtheria/tetanus/pertussis and measles/mumps/rubella vaccines', *The Lancet*, 1995; 345: 567–9.

14. Pollock, T.M., Morris, J. 'A 7-year survey of disorders attributable to vaccination in North West Thames Region', *The Lancet*, 1983; i: 753–7.

15. Committee on Safety of Medicines and the Joint Committee on Vaccination and Immunisation. *Whooping cough.* 1984. HMSO, London.

16. Thompson, N.P., Fleming, D.M., Charlton, J., Ounder, R.E., Wakefield, A.J. 'Social class, ethnicity and smoking in a nationally representative cohort with Crohn's Disease' (Abstract T61), *Gut*, 1996; 39(suppl. 1): A16.

17. Koletzko, S., Sherman, P., Corey, M., Griffiths, A., Smith, C. 'Effect of infant feeding practices on the development of Crohn's disease in childhood', in Atkinson, S.A., Hanson, L.A., Chandra, R.K. (eds) *Breastfeeding, nutrition, infection and infant growth in developed and emerging countries.* 1990. ARTS Biomedical Publishers, St John's, Newfoundland, Canada.

18. Wakefield, A.J., Pittilo, R.M., Sim, R., Cosby, S.L., Stephenson, J.R., Dhillon, A.P. *et al.* 'Evidence of persistent measles virus infection in Crohn's disease', *Journal of Medical Virology*, 1993; 39: 345–53.

19. Ekbom, A., Daszak, P., Kraaz, W., Wakefield, A.J. 'Crohn's disease after in-utero measles virus exposure', *The Lancet*, 1997; 348: 515-7.

20. Lewin, J., Dhillon, A.P., Sim, R., Mazure, G., Pounder, R.E., Wakefield, A.J. 'Persistent measles virus infection of the intestine: confirmation by immunogold electron microscopy', *Gut*, 1995; 36: 564-9.

21. Thompson, N.P., Montgomery, S.M., Pounder, R.E., Wakefield, A.J. 'Is measles vaccination a risk factor for inflammatory bowel disease?', *The Lancet*, 1995; 345: 1071–4.

22. Patriarca, P.A., Beeler, J.A. 'Measles vaccination and inflammatory bowel disease', *The Lancet*, 1995; 345: 1062–3.

23. Farrington, P., Miller, E. 'Measles vaccination as a risk factor for inflammatory bowel disease', *The Lancet*, 1995; 345:1362 (letter).

24. Minor, P.D. 'Measles vaccination as a risk factor for inflammatory bowel disease', *The Lancet*, 1995; 345:1363 (letter).

25. MacDonald, T.T., 'Measles vaccination as a risk factor for inflammatory bowel disease', *The Lancet*, 1995; 345:1363 (letter).

26. Miller, D., Renton, A. 'Measles vaccination as a risk factor for inflammatory bowel disease', *The Lancet*, 1995; 345:1363 (letter).

27. Baxter, T., Radford, J. 'Measles vaccination as a risk factor for inflammatory bowel disease', *The Lancet*, 1995; 345:1363 (letter).

28. Feeney, M., Clegg, A., Winwood, P., Snook, J. for the East Dorset Gastroenterology Group. 'A case-control study of measles vaccination and inflammatory bowel disease', *The Lancet*, 1997; 350: 764-66.

29. Morris, D.L., Montgomery, S.M., Ebrahim, S., Pounder, R.E., Wakefield, A.J. 'Measles vaccination and inflammatory bowel disease in the 1970 cohort study.' *Gut*, 1997; 41 (suppl 3): A37.

30. Gilat, T., Hacohen, D., Lilos, P. and Langman, M.J.S. 'Childhood factors in ulcerative colitis and Crohn's disease: an international co-operative study', *Scandinavian Journal of Gastroenterology*, 1987; 22: 1009-24.

31. Haga, Y., Funakoshi, O., Kuroe, K., Kanazawa, K., Nakajima, H., Saito, H. *et al.* 'Absence of measles viral genomic sequence in intestinal tissues from Crohn's disease by nested polymerase chain reaction', *Gut*, 1996; 38: 211–15.

32. Jones, F., Fine, P., Piracha, S. 'Crohn's disease and measles', *The Lancet*, 1997; 349: 473.

33. Fisher, N.C., Yee, L., Nightingale, P., McEwan, R., Gibson, J.A. 'Measles virus serology in Crohn's disease', *Gut*, 1997; 41: 66-9.

34. Lione, A., Scialli, A.R. 'Perinatal exposure to measles virus and the risk of inflammatory bowel disease', *Reprod Serol*, 1997; 1997: 647-52.

35. Nielsen, L.L.W., Nielsen, N.M., Melbye, M., Sodermann, M., Jacobson, M., Aaby, P. 'Exposure to measles in utero and Crohn's disease: Danish register study', *BMJ*, 1998; 316: 196-7.

36. Metcalf, J. 'Is measles infection associated with Crohn's disease?' *BMJ*, 1998; 516: 186.

37. WHO. 'Expanded programme on immunization (EPI)- association between measles infection and the occurrence of chronic inflammatory bowel disease', *WER*, 1998; 73: 33-40.

38. Afzal, M.A., Minor, P.D., Begley, J., Bentley, M.L., Armitage, E., Ghosh, S., Ferguson, A. 'Absence of measles-virus genome in inflammatory bowel disease', *The Lancet*, 1998; 351: 646-647.

39. Ramsey, M.E.B., Gay, N., Miller, E., Rush, M., White, J., Morgan-Capner, P., Brown, D. 'The epidemiology of measles in England and Wales: rationale for the 1994 national vaccination campaign', *Communicable Disease Report*, 1994; 4(12): R141–R146.

40. Christie, P. 'Measles in Scotland', *Communicable Diseases and Environmental Health in Scotland Weekly Report*, 1994; 28(41): 3-8.

41. Gay, N., Ramsey, M., Cohen, B., Hesketh, L., Morgan-Capner, P., Brown, D., Miller, E. 'The epidemiology of measles in England and Wales since the 1994 vaccination campaign', *Communicable Disease Report*, 1997; 7(R2): R17–21.

42. Cutts, F.T. 'Revaccination against measles and rubella', *British Medical Journal*, 1996; 312: 589–90.

43. Committee on Safety of Medicines; Medicines Control Agency. 'Adverse reactions to measles rubella vaccine', *Current Problems in Pharmacovigilance*, 1995; 21: 9–10.

44. da Silveira, C.M., Salisbury, D.M., de Quadros, C.A. 'Measles vaccination and Guillain-Barré Syndrome, *The Lancet*, 1997; 349: 14-16.

45. Gay, N.J., Miller, E. 'Was a measles epidemic imminent?', *Communicable Disease Report*, 1995; 5: R204–R207.

46. Department of Health. *Immunisation against infectious disease*. 1996. HMSO, London.

47. Jones, A.G.H., White, J.M., Begg, N.T. 'The impact of MMR vaccine on mumps infection in England and Wales', *Communicable Disease Report*, 1991; 1(9): R93–R96.

48. Sosin, D.M., Cochi, S.L., Gunn, R.A., Jennings, C.E., Preblud, S.R. 'Changing epidemiology of mumps and its impact on university campuses', *Pediatrics*, 1989; 84: 779–84.

49. American Academy of Pediatrics, Committee on Infectious Diseases. *Red Book*. 1994. American Academy of Pediatrics, Illinois.

50. Miller, E., Goldacre, M., Pugh, S., Colville, A., Farrington, P., Flower, A. *et al.* 'Risk of aseptic meningitis after measles, mumps and rubella vaccine in UK children', *The Lancet*, 1993; 341: 979–82.

51. Plotkin, S.A., Mortimer, E.A. (eds) 'Rubella vaccine', *Vaccines*, 1994. W.B. Saunders, Philadelphia.

52. Bakshi, S.S., Cooper, L.Z. 'Rubella and mumps vaccines', in Pediatric Vaccinations: Update 1990. *Pediatric Clinics of North America*, 1990; 37(3): 651–68.

53. Bayer, W.L., Sherman, F.E., Michaels, P.H., Szeto, I.L.F., Lewis, J.H. 'Purpura in congenital and acquired rubella', *The New England Journal of Medicine*, 1965; 273: 1362–6.

54. Miller, E., Cradock-Watson, J.E., Pollock, T.M. 'Consequences of confirmed rubella at successive stages of pregnancy', *The Lancet*, 1982; i: 871–4.

55. Howson, P., Howe, C.J. and Fineberg, H. V. (eds) *Adverse effects of pertussis and rubella vaccines*. 1991. National Academy Press, Washington.

56. Slater, P.E., Ben-Zvi, T., Fogel, A., Ehrenfeld, M., Ever-Hadani, S. 'Absence of an association between rubella vaccination and arthritis in underimmune postpartum women', *Vaccine*, 1995; 13 (16): 1529-31.

57. Ray, P., Black, S., Shinefield, H., Dillon, A., Schwalbe, J., Holmes, S., Hadler, S., Chen, R., Cochi, S., Wassilak, S., for the Vaccine Safety Datalink Team. 'Risk of chronic arthropathy among women after rubella vaccination', *JAMA*, 1997; 278: 551-6.

58. Tingle, A.J., Mitchell, L.A., Grace, M., Middleton, P., Mathias, R., MacWilliam, L., Chalmers, A. 'Randomised double-blind placebo-controlled study on adverse effects of rubella immunisation in seronegative women', *The Lancet*, 1997; 349: 1277-81.

59. Jonville-Bera, A.P., Autret, E., Galy-Eyraud, C., Hessel, L. 'Thrombocytopenic purpura after measles, mumps and rubella vaccination: a retrospective survey by the French Regional Pharmacovigilance Centres and Pasteur-Mérieux Sérums et Vaccins', *Pediatric Infectious Disease Journal*, 1996; 15: 44–8.

60. Tookey, P.A., Jones, G., Miller, B.H.R., Peckham, C.S. 'Rubella vaccination in pregnancy', *Communicable Disease Report*, 1991; 1: R86–R88.

61. Miller, E. 'Rubella in the United Kingdom', *Epidemiology and Infection*, 1991; 107:31–42.

62. Miller, E., Tookey, P., Morgan-Capner, P., Hesketh, L., Brown, D., Waight, P. *et al.* 'Rubella surveillance to June 1994: third joint report from the PHLS and the National Congenital Rubella Surveillance Programme', *Communicable Disease Report*, 1994; 4: R146–R152.

63. Markowitz, L.E., Katz, S.L. 'Measles vaccine,' in Plotkin, S.A., Mortimer, E.A. (eds.) *Vaccines*, 1994. W.B. Saunders, Philadelphia.

64. White, J.M., Leon, S. 'COVER (Cover of vaccination evaluated rapidly): 34', *Communicable Disease Report*, 1995; 5: R105–R106.

65. Issacs, D., Menser, M. 'Measles, mumps, rubella, and varicella', *The Lancet*, 1990; 335: 1384–7.

66. Kanner, L. 'Autistic disturbances of affective contact', *Nervous child*, 1943; 2: 217-50.

67. *Diagnostic and statistical manual of mental disorders*. 4th edn. 1994. American Psychiatric Association, Washington DC.

68. Gillberg, C., Coleman, M. *The biology of the autistic syndromes*. 2nd edn. 1992. MacKeith Press, London.

69. Bolton, P., MacDonald, H., Pickles, A., Rios, P., Goode, S., Crowson, M., Bailey A., Rutter, M. 'A case control family history study of autism.' *J Child Psychol and Psychiat*, 1994; 33: 877-900.

70. Bailey, A., Le Couteur, A., Gottesman, I., Bolton, P., Simonoff, E., Yuzda, E., Rutter, M. 'Autism as a strongly genetic disorder: evidence from a British twin study', *Psychol Med* 1995; 25: 63-77.

71. Chess, S.J. 'Follow-up report on autism in congenital rubella', *Autism Childhood Schiz*, 1977; 7: 69-81.

72. Laxer, G., Rey, M., Ritvo, E.R. 'A comparison of potentially pathologic factors in European children with autism, Down's syndrome, and multiple physical handicaps', *J Autism Develop Dis*, 1988; 18: 309-313.

73. Wing, L. *The autistic spectrum. A guide for parents and professionals*. 1996. Constable, London.

74. Wakefield, A.J., Murch, S.H., Anthony, A., Linnell, J., Casson, D.M., Malik, M., Berelowitz, M., Dhillon, A.P., Thompson, M.A., Harvey, P., Valentine, A., Davies, S.E., Walker-Smith, J.A. 'Ileal-lymphoid nodular hyperplasia, non-specific colitis, and pervasive developmental disorder in children', *The Lancet*, 1998; 351: 637-641.

75. Chen, R.T., DeStefano, F. 'Vaccine adverse events: causal or coincidental?' *The Lancet*, 1998; 351: 611-612.

76. Shapiro, E.D., Ward, J.I. 'The epidemiology and prevention of disease caused by *Haemophilus influenzae* type b', *Epidemiologic Reviews*, 1991; 13: 113–42.

77. Bedford, H., Peckham, C., Halket, S., Hurley, R., Harvey, D., de Louvois, J. 'National follow up of *Haemophilus influenzae* meningitis' (letter), *Archives of Disease in Childhood*, 1993; 69: 711–12.

78. Booy, R., Moxon, E.R. 'Prevention of *Haemophilus influenzae* type b infection by immunisation', *Current Paediatrics*, 1993; 3: 20–3.

79. Scheibner, V. *Vaccination – 100 years of orthodox research shows that vaccines represent a medical assault on the immune system*. 1993. Australian Print Group, Victoria.

80. Neustaedter, R. 'The immunization decision', *The Family Health Series*. 1990. North Atlantic Books, Berkeley.

81. Ward, J.I., Broome, C.V., Harrison, L.H., Shinefield, H., Black, S. '*Haemophilus influenzae* type b vaccines: lessons for the future', *Pediatrics*, 1988; 81(6): 886–93.

82. Booy, R., Hodgson, S., Carpenter, L., Mayon-White, R.T., Slack, M.P.E., Macfarlane, J.A. *et al*. 'Efficacy of *Haemophilus influenzae* type b conjugate vaccine PRP-T', *The Lancet*, 1994; 344: 362–6.

83. Goldblatt, D., Fairley, C.K., Cartwright, K., Miller, E. 'Interchangeability of conjugated *Haemophilus influenzae* type b vaccines during primary immunisation of infants', *British Medical Journal*, 1996; 312: 817–18.

84. Begg, N.T. *et al*. 'Antibody responses and symptoms after DTP and either tetanus or diphtheria *Haemophilus influenzae* type b conjugate vaccines given for primary immunisation by separate or mixed injection', *Vaccine*, 1995; 13(16): 1547–50.

85. Booy, R., Taylor, S.A., Dobson, S.R.M., Issacs, D., Sleight, G., Aitken, S. *et al*. 'Immunogenicity and safety of PRP-T conjugate vaccine given according to the British accelerated immunisation schedule', *Archives of Disease in Childhood*, 1992; 67: 475–8.

86. Heath, P., Booy, R., Slack, M., Begg, N.T., Griffiths, H., Anderson, E. *et al*. 'Invasive *Haemophilus influenzae* infection following Hib immunisation'. *Proceedings of British Paediatric Association Annual Meeting 1995*; 67: 24.

87. Peltola, H., Kilpi, T., Anttila, M. 'Rapid disappearance of *Haemophilus influenzae* type b meningitis after routine childhood immunisation with conjugate vaccines', *The Lancet*, 1992; 340: 592–4.

88. Adams, W.G., Deaver, K.A., Cochi, S.L., Plikaytis, B.D., Zell, E.R., Broome, C.V. *et al*. 'Decline of childhood *Haemophilus influenzae* type b (Hib) disease in the Hib vaccine era', *Journal of the American Medical Association*, 1993; 269(2): 221–6.

89. Department of Health. PL CMO (94)2. *Meningococcal infection: meningitis and septicaemia*. 1994. HMSO, London.

90. Ross, E. 'Childhood immunization', in Harvey, D., Miles, M., Smyth, D. (eds) *Community child health and paediatrics*. 1995. Butterworth-Heinemann, Oxford.

91. Miller, E., Vurdien, J.E., White, J.M. 'The epidemiology of pertussis in England and Wales', *Communicable Disease Report*, 1992; 2: R152–R154.

92. Cherry, J.D. 'Acellular pertussis vaccines – a solution to the pertussis problem', *The Journal of Infectious Diseases*, 1993; 168: 21–4.

93. Williams, W.O., Kwantes, W., Joynson, D.H.M. 'Effect of low pertussis vaccination uptake on a large community', *British Medical Journal*, 1981; 282: 23.

94. Mortimer, E.A. 'Pertussis vaccines', in Plotkin, S.A., Mortimer E.A. (eds) *Vaccines*. 1994. W.B. Saunders, Philadelphia.

95. Mark, A., Granstrom, M. 'Impact of pertussis on the afflicted child and family', *Pediatric Infectious Disease Journal*, 1992; 11: 554–7.

96. Grob, P.R., Crowder, M.J., Robbins, J.F. 'Effect of vaccination on severity and dissemination of whooping cough', *British Medical Journal*, 1981; 282: 1925–8.

97. Jenkinson, D. 'Natural course of 500 consecutive cases of whooping cough: a general practice population study', *British Medical Journal*, 1995; 310: 299–302.

98. Rouse, A.M. 'Estimating the chance of an inadequately immunised child getting pertussis', *Public Health*, 1992; 106: 155–62.

99. Binkin, N.J., Samaso, S., Tozzi, A.E., Scuderi, G., Greco, D. & D. 'Epidemiology of pertussis in a developed country with low vaccination coverage: the Italian experience', *Pediatric Infectious Disease Journal*, 1992; 11: 653–61.

100. PHLS Epidemiological Research Laboratory and 21 Area Health Authorities. 'Efficacy of pertussis vaccine in England', *British Medical Journal*, 1982; 285: 357–9.

101. Miller, C.L., Fletcher, W.B. 'Severity of notified whooping cough', *British Medical Journal*, 1976; 1: 117–19.

102. McKendrick, M.W., Gully, P.R., Geddes, A.M. 'Protection against pertussis by immunisation', *British Medical Journal*, 1980; 281: 1390–1.

103. Heininger, U., Cherry, J.D., Eckhardt, T., Lorenz, C., Christenson, P., Stehr, K. 'Clinical and laboratory diagnosis of pertussis in the regions of a large vaccine efficacy trial in Germany', *Pediatric Infectious Disease Journal*, 1993; 12: 504–9.

104. Golden, G.S. 'Pertussis vaccine and injury to the brain', *The Journal of Pediatrics*, 1990; 116(6): 854–61.

105. Baxter, D.N. 'Pertussis immunisation of children with histories of neurological problems', *British Medical Journal*, 1994; 309: 1619.

106. Miller, D., Wadsworth, J., Ross, E. 'Severe neurological illness. Further analysis of the British National Childhood Encephalopathy Study', *Tokai Journal of Experimental and Clinical Medicine*, 1988; 13: 145–55.

107. Kulenkampff, M.M., Schwartzman, J.S., Wilson, J. 'Neurological complications of pertussis inoculation', *Archives of Disease in Childhood*, 1974; 49: 46–9.

108. Miller, E., Jacombs, B., Pollock, T.M. 'Whooping cough notifications' (letter), *British Medical Journal*, 1980; 1: 718.

109. Nottingham Health Authority. *Vaccination training procedure manual for trainers*. 3rd edn. 1988. Nottingham Health Authority, Nottingham.

110. Stuart-Smith, S. *Judgment in Loveday vs Renton & Wellcome*. Royal Courts of Justice, London, 29–30 March 1988.

111. Cody, C.L., Baraff, L.J., Cherry, J.D., Marcy, S.M., Manclark, C.R. 'Nature and rate of adverse reactions associated with DTP and DT immunizations in infants and children', *Pediatrics*, 1981; 68: 650–60.

112. Walker, A.M., Jick, H., Perera, D.R., Knauss, T.A., Thompson, R.S. 'Neurologic events following diphtheria-tetanus-pertussis immunization', *Pediatrics*, 1988; 81: 345–9.

113. Gale, J.L., Thapa, P.B., Wassilak, S.G.F. *et al.* 'Risk of serious acute neurological illness after immunization with diphtheria-tetanus-pertussis vaccine', *Journal of the American Medical Association*, 1994; 271: 37–41.

114. Elliman, D.A.C. 'Pertussis immunisation and serious neurological illness in children', *Maternal and Child Health*, 1994; November: 351–3.

115. Blennow, M., Granstrom, M., Jaatmaa, E., Olin, P. 'Primary immunization of infants with an acellular pertussis vaccine in double-blind randomized clinical trial', *Pediatrics*, 1988; 82: 293–9.

116. Miller, E. *et al.* 'Phase II trial of whole-cell pertussis vaccine vs an acellular vaccine containing agglutinogens', *The Lancet*, 1991; 337: 70–3.

117. Kimura, M., Kuno-Sakai, H. 'Pertussis vaccines in Japan', *Acta Paediatrica Japonica*, 1988; 30: 143–53.

118. Greco, D., Salmaso, S., Mastrantonio, P., Giuliano, M., Tozzi, A.E., Anemona, A. *et al.* 'A controlled trial of two acellular vaccines and one whole-cell vaccine against pertussis', *The New England Journal of Medicine*, 1996; 334(6): 341–8.

119. Gustafsson, L., Hallander, H.O., Olin, P., Reizenstein, E., Storsaeter, J. 'A controlled trial of a two-component acellular, a five-component acellular, and a whole-cell pertussis vaccine', *The New England Journal of Medicine*, 1996; 334(6): 349–55.

120. Miller, E., Ashworth, L.A., Redhead, K., Thornton, C., Waight, P.A., Coleman, T. 'Effect of schedule on reactogenecity and antibody persistence of acellular and whole-cell pertussis vaccines: value of laboratory tests as predictors of clinical performance', *Vaccine*, 1997; 15: 51-60.

121. Center for Disease Control. 'FDA approval of a second acellular pertussis vaccine for use among infants and young children', *Morbidity and Mortality Weekly Report* 1997; 46(5): 110-111.

122. Schmitt-Grohé, Cherry, J.D., Heininger, U., Überall, M.A., Pineda, E., Stehr, K. 'Pertussis in German adults', *Clin Inf Dis*, 1995; 21: 860-6.

123. Nenning, M.E., Shinefield, H.R., Edwards, K.M., Black, S.B., Fireman, B.H. 'Prevalence and incidence of adult pertussis in an urban population', *JAMA*, 1996; 275: 1672-4.

124. Ramsey, M.E.B., Begg, N.T., Gandhi, J., Brown, D. 'Antibody response and viral excretion after live polio vaccine or a combined schedule of live and inactivated polio vaccines', *Pediatric Infectious Disease Journal*, 1994; 13: 1117–21.

125. Patriarca, P.A., Foege, W.H., Swartz, T.A. 'Progress in polio eradication', *The Lancet*, 1993; 342: 1461–4.

126. Oostvogel, P.M., van Wijngaarden, J.K., van der Avoort, H.G.A.M., Mulders, M.N., Conyn van Spaaendonck, M.A.E., Rumke, H.C. *et al.* 'Poliomyelitis outbreak in an unvaccinated community in the Netherlands, 1992–93', *The Lancet*, 1994; 344: 665–70.

127. Joce, R., Wood, D., Brown, D., Begg, N.T. 'Paralytic poliomyelitis in England and Wales, 1985–91', *British Medical Journal*, 1992; 305: 79–82.

128. Sweet, B.H., Hilleman, M.R. 'The vacuolating virus SV40', *Proc Soc Exp Biol Med*, 1960; 105: 420-427.

129. Eddy, B.E. 'Simian virus (SV40): An oncogenic virus', *Prog Exp Tumor Res*, 1964; 4: 1-26.

130. Gerber, P., Hottle, G.A., Grubbs, R.E. 'Inactivation of vacuolating virus (SV40) by formaldehyde', *Proc Soc Exp Biol Med*, 1961; 108: 205-209.

131. Bergsagel, D.J., Finegold, M.J., Butel, J.S., Kupsky, W.J., Garcea, R.L. 'DNA sequences similar to those of simian virus 40 in ependymomas and choroid plexus tumors of childhood', *N Engl J Med*, 1992: 326: 988-993.

132. Martini, F., Iaccheri, L., Lazzarin, L., Carinci, P., Corallini, A., Gerosa, M., Iuzzolino, P., Barbanti-Brodano, G., Tognon, M. 'SV40 early region and large T antigen in human brain tumors, peripheral blood cells, and sperm fluids from healthy individuals', *Cancer Res*, 1996; 56 (20): 4820-4825.

133. Carbone, M., Rizzo, P., Procopio, A., Giuliano, M., Gebhardt, M.C., Mangham, C., Hansen, M., Malkin, D.F., Bushart, G., Pompetti, F., Picci, P., Levine, A.S., Bergsagel, J.D., Garcea, R.L. 'SV40-like sequence in human bone tumors', *Oncogene*, 1996; 13 (3): 527-535.

134. Strickler, H.D., Goedert, J.J., Fleming, M., Travis, W.D., Williams, A.E., Rabkin, C.S., Daniel, R.W., Shah, K.V. 'Simian virus 40 and pleural mesothelioma in humans', *Cancer Epidemiology, Biomarkers & Prevention*, 1996; 5: 473-5.

135. Geissler, F., Scherneek, S., Prokoph, H., Zimmerman, W., Staneczek, W. 'SV40 in human brain tumors: Risk factor or passenger?' In Giraldo, G., Beth, E. (eds). *The role of viruses in human cancer*. Vol. 2. 1984. Elsevier, New York.

136. Strickler, H.D., Rosenberg, P.S., Devesa, S.S., Hertel, J., Fraumeni, J.F., Goedert, J.J. 'Contamination of poliovirus vaccine with simian virus 40 (1955-63) and subsequent cancer rates', *JAMA*, 1998; 279 (4): 292-295.

137. Cherry, J. 'Polio', in *Childhood immunisation state of the art. Conference proceedings*. 1995. King's College, London.

138. World Health Organization. *Global programme for vaccines and immunization. Programme report 1994.* 1995. WHO/GPV/95.1.

139. James, W. *Immunization – the reality behind the myth.* 1988. Bergin & Garvey, New York.

140. Dudgeon, J.A., Cutting, W.A.M. (eds) *Immunization: principles and practice.* 1991. Chapman & Hall Medical, London.

141. Leese, B., Bosanquet, N. 'Immunization in the UK: policy review and future economic options', *Vaccine*, 1992; 10(8): 491–9.

142. Communicable Disease Surveillance Centre. 'A case of diphtheria from Pakistan', *Communicable Disease Report*, 1994; 4: 37.

143. Center for Disease Control. 'Diphtheria epidemic – new independent states of the former Soviet Union, 1990–1994', *Morbidity and Mortality Weekly Report*, 1995; 44(10): 177–81.

144. Begg, N.T., Balraj, V. 'Diphtheria: are we ready for it?', *Archives of Disease in Childhood*, 1995: 73: 568–72.

145. Maple, P.A., Efstratiou, A., George, R.C., Andrews, N.J., Sesardic, D. 'Diphtheria immunity in UK blood donors', *The Lancet*, 1995; 345: 963–5.

146. Cumberland, N.S., Kidd, A.G., Karalliedde, L. 'Immunity to tetanus in United Kingdom populations', *Journal of Infection*, 1993; 27: 255–60.

147. Clarke, A., Rudd, P. 'Neonatal BCG immunisation', *Archives of Disease in Childhood*, 1992; 67: 473–4.

148. Watson, J.M., Fern, K.J., Porter, J.D.H., Whitmore, S.E. 'Notifications of tuberculosis in England and Wales, 1982–1989', *Communicable Disease Report*, 1991; 1: R13–R16.

149. Watson, J.M. 'Tuberculosis in Britain today', *British Medical Journal*, 1993; 306: 221–2.

150. Conway, S.P. 'BCG vaccination in children', *British Medical Journal*, 1990; 301: 1059–60.

151. Citron, K.M. 'BCG vaccination against tuberculosis: international perspectives', *British Medical Journal*, 1993; 306: 222–3.

152. Packe, G.E., Innes, J.A. 'Protective effect of BCG vaccination in infant Asians: a case-control study', *Archives of Disease in Childhood*, 1988; 63: 277–81.

153. Curtis, H.M., Leck, I., Bamford, F.N. 'Incidence of childhood tuberculosis after neonatal BCG vaccination', *The Lancet*, 1984; i: 145–8.

154. Price, J.F. 'BCG vaccination', *Archives of Disease in Childhood*, 1982; 57: 485–6.

155. Moradpour, D., Wands, J.R. 'Understanding hepatitis B virus infection', *The New England Journal of Medicine*, 1995; 332(16): 1092–3.

156. Eddleston, A. 'Hepatitis', *The Lancet*, 1990; 335: 1142–5.

157. Teo, C.G. 'The virology and serology of hepatitis: an overview', *Communicable Disease Review*, 1992; 2(10): R109–R114.

158. Smith, C.P., Parle, M., Morris, D.J. 'Implementation of government recommendations for immunising infants at risk of hepatitis B', *British Medical Journal*, 1994; 309: 1339.

159. Viral Hepatitis Prevention Board. *Viral hepatitis.* 1996. Viral Hepatitis Prevention Board, Antwerp.

160. Krugman, S., Stevens, C.E. 'Hepatitis B vaccine', in Plotkin, S.A., Mortimer, E.A. (eds) *Vaccines.* 1994. W.B. Saunders, Philadelphia.

161. Margolis, H.S. 'Prevention of acute and chronic liver disease through immunization: hepatitis B and beyond', *The Journal of Infectious Diseases*, 1993; 168: 9–14.

162. Niu, M.T., Davis, D.M., Ellenberg, S. 'Recombinant hepatitis B vaccination of neonates and infants: emerging safety data from the Vaccine Adverse Event Reporting Systems', *Pediatric Infectious Disease Journal*, 1996: 15(9): 771–6.

163. Committee on Infectious Diseases. 'Universal hepatitis B immunization', *Pediatrics*, 1992; 89: 795–800.

164. US Preventive Services Task Force. *Guide to clinical preventive services.* 1996. International Medical Publishing, Inc., Alexandria, Virginia.

165. Forrest, J.M., Burgess, M.A. 'Update on immunization'. *Current Opinion in Pediatrics*, 1996; 8: 21–7.

166. Bellanti, J.A. 'Basic immunologic principles underlying vaccination procedures', *Pediatric Clinics of North America*, 1990; 37(3): 513–30.

167. Brown, F. 'From Jenner to genes – the new vaccines', *The Lancet*, 1990; 335: 587–90.